Practice guideline development manual

College of Occupational Therapists

Third edition 2017

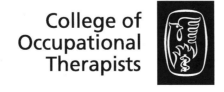

College of
Occupational
Therapists

3rd edition published in 2017
by the College of Occupational Therapists Ltd
106–114 Borough High Street
London SE1 1LB
www.cot.org.uk

First published in Great Britain in 2004 by the College of Occupational Therapists
Second edition published in 2011 and reprinted with amendments in 2014
This third edition supersedes all previous editions

Copyright © College of Occupational Therapists 2017

Editors: Mandy Sainty, Research and Development Manager, and Julia Roberts, Quality
Programme Manager, on behalf of the College of Occupational Therapists
Category: Practice Guidelines
Date for Review: 2022

Other enquiries about this document should be addressed to the Professional Practice
Department at the above address.

British Library Cataloguing in Publication Data
A catalogue record for this book is available from the British Library

ISBN 978 1 905944 61 3

Typeset by Servis Filmsetting Ltd, Stockport, Cheshire
Digitally printed on demand in Great Britain by the Lavenham Press, Suffolk

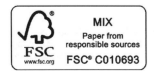

Contents

Foreword   v

1   Introduction   1

2   About practice guidelines   2
    2.1 Defining occupational therapy practice guidelines   2
    2.2 Characteristics of high-quality practice guidelines   2
    2.3 Practitioner responsibilities   3

3   Guideline development   4
    3.1   Selecting a topic   4
    3.2   The guideline development group   5
    3.3   Stakeholder involvement   6
    3.4   Service user and carer involvement   8
    3.5   Scope and purpose of the guideline   9
    3.6   Developing the clinical, healthcare or social practice questions   10
    3.7   Finding the supporting knowledge and evidence   11
    3.8   Appraising the evidence   13
    3.9   Grading quality of evidence – GRADE   15
    3.10 Formulating and grading recommendations   17
    3.11 Strength and overall grading of recommendations   19
    3.12 Writing the guideline   20
    3.13 Peer review   20
    3.14 Review and updating   21
    3.15 Funding mechanisms for guideline development   22
    3.16 Conflicts of interest   22
    3.17 Decision-making processes   23

4   Implementation of guidelines   24
    4.1 Selecting implementation techniques and support tools   24

5   The College's appraisal and approval process   26
    5.1 Practice Publications Group   26
    5.2 Guideline appraisal   26
    5.3 Guideline development timeline   26
    5.4 Proposal stage (3–5 months)   27
    5.5 Development stage (11–13 months)   30
    5.6 Approval and publication stage (3–4 months)   33
    5.7 Post-publication stage   34

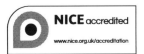

NICE has accredited the process used by the College of Occupational Therapists to produce its practice guidelines. Accreditation is valid for five years from January 2013 and is applicable to guidance produced using the processes described in the *Practice guideline development manual* 3rd edition (2017). More information on accreditation can be viewed at *www.nice.org.uk/accreditation*

Contents

Appendices

1	Proposal form for the PPG	38
2	Scope form for the PPG	43
3	Scope stakeholder information	47
4	Appraisal tools	49
5	Evidence tables template	50
6	Recommendation decision table template	51
7	Guideline document template	52
8	Peer review proforma	55
9	Conflicts of interest declaration form	57
10	Management of conflicts of interest	59
11	The College's Practice Publications Group terms of reference	61
12	College resources for guideline developers	64
13	Guideline development group responsibilities	66
14	Copyright	68
15	Summary chart of key stages of guideline development	69

References 70

Foreword

Occupational therapy practice guidelines are crucial for the development of innovative and evidence-informed practice which describes the unique contribution of occupational therapy to the health and wellbeing of service users. They also serve as an audit tool to facilitate improvement of the quality of occupational therapy services, all of which is important for future business planning and commissioning of occupational therapy.

Since the publication of the last edition of this manual in 2011, the College's process for developing guidelines was accredited by NICE in January 2013, making us eligible to use the NICE Accreditation mark on our published guidelines. This was a commendable achievement, as COT was the first Allied Health Profession to achieve NICE Accreditation. Guidelines developed following the College's NICE Accredited process are eligible to be considered as sources of evidence by NICE when developing Quality Standards, and the published guidelines are profiled within NICE Evidence Search, which is available to all.

I would like to congratulate the authors on this 3rd edition of the *Practice guideline development manual*. The College has recognised the need to ensure guideline development groups have the best possible information to support them in their guideline project, and that the rigorous process is adequately described against the criteria required for NICE Accreditation. Whilst the guideline development process itself has not changed, this edition provides additional details and clarity around a number of key areas such as conflicts of interest; stakeholder involvement, including service users' and carers' input in the guidelines development process; decision-making; and post-publication activities. This comprehensive, detailed document clearly articulates guideline development in a step-by-step process through the proposal; development; approval and publication; and post-publication stages.

Of course, the development of guidelines using the COT process would not be possible without the expertise, significant commitment and contribution of individual COT members, the support of COT Specialist Sections, and the positive engagement of a variety of stakeholders and service users. To date, five guidelines have been developed and published using the COT accredited process and another one is currently under development, scheduled for publication in September 2017.

We all have a duty to promote occupational therapy and raise our profile with key stakeholders. The development of practice guidelines enables us to do this, building a robust base of evidence to further the profession. So whether it is contributing to a guideline development group, applying the evidence within the guidelines to inform your practice, or using the contents to influence business planning and commissioning processes, on behalf of the profession, I encourage you to get involved.

I am sure you will enjoy engaging with this valuable and rewarding activity.

Dr Patricia McClure
Chair of Council, College of Occupational Therapists

1 Introduction

The College of Occupational Therapists (COT) is the professional body and voluntary membership organisation for occupational therapists throughout the United Kingdom. It is a subsidiary of and trading name for the British Association of Occupational Therapists (BAOT) which also acts as a trade union. The College sets the professional and educational standards for the occupational therapy profession and represents the profession at national and international levels. In addition, eleven College of Occupational Therapists Specialist Sections support expert clinical practice.

The College is committed to supporting therapists in developing evidence-based practice guidelines to underpin their practice. This manual provides the structure and process to guide its members who wish to develop profession-specific guidelines for publication by the College of Occupational Therapists. It aims to ensure that the practice guideline development process is not only tailored to the occupational therapy profession and its specific needs, but is also robust, rigorous and sustainable for the future.

Practice guidelines published by the College are publicly available from the College's website (*www.cot.org.uk*).

How to use this manual

Section 1   Introduction
This section outlines the value and importance of practice guidelines.

Section 2   About practice guidelines
This section defines practice guidelines and their characteristics, including legal implications. It is essential background reading to help occupational therapists understand how guidelines can support their practice.

Section 3   Guideline development
This section will equip the reader with the basic knowledge and understanding required to get involved in developing guidelines. It provides a comprehensive guide to the different components and methodologies used to ensure a rigorous and robust practice guideline development process. Those wishing to develop guidelines in partnership with the College must also read section 5 for specific step-by-step details.

Section 4   Implementation of guidelines
Areas to consider in order to help implement guidelines effectively are outlined in this section.

Section 5   The College's appraisal and approval process
Specific information relevant to guideline development groups wishing to work in partnership with the College is provided in this section. For ease of reading, the information is cross-referenced back to the relevant stages contained within section 3.

Appendices
Additional supporting material referred to in sections 2–5, including example forms and templates, which will be used within the process.

2 About practice guidelines

2.1 Defining occupational therapy practice guidelines

Guidelines define the best and most effective practice for a specific area of occupational therapy, condition, population and/or set of circumstances. Guidelines are systematically developed recommendations based on the best available evidence and knowledge, or a consensus of expert opinion. They assist the occupational therapist in their decision-making about appropriate interventions, and describe the profession's contribution within a given care pathway. A guideline should always allow for professional or clinical judgement.

> **Key points: The value of occupational therapy practice guidelines**
>
> • To support evidence-informed practice.
>
> • To support business planning and commissioning by describing the unique contribution of occupational therapy.
>
> • To improve the quality of occupational therapy services by facilitating audit against guideline recommendations.

2.2 Characteristics of high-quality practice guidelines

The framework that underpins the College's guideline development process is based on the 25 criteria used by the NICE Accreditation Programme (National Institute for Health and Care Excellence (NICE) 2014, pp40–42). An accredited standard of guideline development provides assurance that the recommendations have been robustly developed, are fit for purpose, and that their application in practice will facilitate the delivery of improved outcomes.

> **Key points: Core elements of a quality guideline**
>
> • A clear scope and purpose concerned with the overall aim of the guidance, the specific health and wellbeing questions and the target population.
>
> • Stakeholder involvement to ensure that the guidance represents the views of its intended users and those affected by the recommendations.
>
> • Use of a rigorous and systematic process to appraise and synthesise the evidence and to develop recommendations, giving due consideration to benefits and risks.
>
> • A clearly presented format, using unambiguous language appropriate to the specified target audience.
>
> • Application of the guideline which includes the consideration of barriers, cost implications and approaches to support implementation.
>
> • Evidence of a transparent process that demonstrates editorial independence.

2.3 Practitioner responsibilities

The existence and use of guidelines does not remove the responsibility and duty of care placed upon the occupational therapist.

Routine professional activity, such as record keeping, risk management and safeguarding confidentiality, is every practitioner's responsibility. Adherence to regulatory and professional body requirements is assumed and therefore is not covered specifically in practice guidelines.

Practitioners are responsible for ensuring that the interpretation of guidelines is appropriate to the situation, taking into consideration the individualised needs of the service user, local influences, as well as social and/or cultural practices. If the practitioner should decide that it is appropriate to deviate from a practice guideline, this should be recorded in the service user's records, along with the rationale for the decision made.

There may be circumstances in which there is more than one guideline for a given condition or situation, possibly giving conflicting recommendations. The final decision on the best intervention or action always depends upon the clinical reasoning and judgement of the professional, in shared decision-making with the service user and multidisciplinary team, as appropriate.

3 Guideline development

All guidelines published by the College must follow the process described in this manual as accredited by NICE.

3.1 Selecting a topic

Topics for inclusion in occupational therapy practice guidelines can be initiated by College groups, its Specialist Sections or members.

Key points: Selecting a topic

There are a number of key questions to consider when selecting a topic:

- Why is this particular guideline needed at this particular time?

- Is there sufficient occupational therapy evidence to support the development of a guideline in this topic area?

- Are there significant or unexplained variations in practice, which could be improved?

- Is the potential subject high volume, high risk or high cost to service providers and users?

- What are the cost implications of the development and implementation work of the potential guideline?

- Is the topic an area that has gained interest and therefore may gain local or national funding and support for the development and implementation work?

- Is there evidence or a consensus of expert opinion to identify best practice?

- Is the investment of time and money in the development of the guideline likely to be repaid by real changes and benefits in the health and social care provided?

- Is the topic important in terms of the process and outcomes of occupational therapy?

- Can the topic be clearly defined to avoid being too broad in scope?

- Will change benefit the service user or carers?

The College uses these questions and others as a basis to inform its decision as to whether to support the development and publication of a practice guideline.

The flowcharts in section 5 identify the typical process for guidelines developed in partnership with the College. Parties interested in developing national occupational therapy guidelines are encouraged to contact the College before progressing with a project. This can facilitate collaborative working and avoid duplication of activity on similar topics.

3.2 The guideline development group

A guideline development group is a recognised method by which practice guidelines can be developed. This approach enables the responsibility for the work to be shared, maximises use of the expertise of different members, and encourages broader ownership of the resulting guideline. The group must ensure that it is self-sufficient in terms of the skills required to develop the proposed publication.

Key points: The guideline development group

The following should be considered:

- Will the publication be best produced in collaboration with another professional body or organisation or is another organisation already engaged in similar work?

- What involvement of service users and carers will be established?

- How will a range of stakeholders be involved?

- Are those who will be influential in implementing and using the guideline involved?

- How many are in the group? A core group of 6-8 allows sufficient breadth of expertise whilst remaining a manageable, functional group.

- Does the core group have members with the relevant skills, or have access to the following:

  - project lead (chair, facilitate and project-manage),

  - editorial lead (writing for publication),

  - expert/experienced practitioners,

  - evidence/research skills (evidence searching, critical appraisal),

  - guideline awareness or development,

  - lay representatives/service users, i.e. 'experts by experience',

  - administrative support?

- Does the core group have access to individuals who will be able to support the appraisal process or provide other co-opted expertise/advice via a reference group?

- Do group members have access to libraries or higher education institutions?

- Do all potential members have the time available and support from their employers, if necessary?

- How will an inclusive approach to participation be facilitated (for example, accessible environments, teleconferencing)?

- Has the responsibility for reviewing and updating the published guideline been discussed and the process agreed?

The guidelines will have greater credibility if the development group represents and/or engages with a wide range of appropriate stakeholders, lay representatives, service users and those who will have some responsibility for implementing the recommendations. Not all contributors or stakeholders will necessarily need to be involved at all stages of the process or for the full term of the guideline development project. Some contributors can be co-opted as and when their relevant expertise is required.

The process defined in this manual relates to the development of profession-specific guidelines, i.e. the target audience is occupational therapists. Representatives of the profession are therefore likely to make up the majority of the core guideline development group. Ideally this should include representation from the four UK nations and from practice, research and education. This ensures that a balance of perspectives can be brought to a project.

The group will need to have a strategy or plan for the development of the proposed guideline. Details such as the rationale, guideline group skill mix, stakeholder involvement, market context, and support and funding will need to be detailed within the College's proposal form (Appendix 1). A two-year timeline, which includes the stages outlined in this process manual, must also be completed. This will enable members to have a realistic idea of the commitment required and will help the group maintain a momentum. The project lead will be the link to the College throughout the development and publication process.

3.3 Stakeholder involvement

Whilst the core guideline development group membership will predominantly be occupational therapists, stakeholder involvement is integral to the development of high-quality practice guidelines.

> **Stakeholders are defined as follows:**
>
> *Professional organisations and bodies:* e.g. other Allied Health Professions (AHPs), medical organisations, Royal College of Nursing (RCN), British Association of Social Workers (BASW), charitable or third sector organisations, commissioners.
>
> *Lay people:* i.e. individuals or organisations representing and/or supporting service users or carers.
>
> *Service users and carers:* i.e. people who use or have used occupational therapy services.
>
> *End users:* i.e. occupational therapists in all work settings who will use the guideline.

The rationale for collaboration with stakeholders in the development of a guideline who are not occupational therapists is multifarious, but includes:

• Representatives from different organisations/backgrounds can facilitate a wider discussion of the issues in relation to a guideline topic.

• Health and social care professionals (often via professional bodies or multi-agency representatives working with service user groups in the given specialism) can provide a viewpoint based on their clinical expertise and knowledge, within the context of multidisciplinary/multi-agency working.

• Organisations or groups representing service users, and individual service users and carers, can draw on key experiences and expectations from the 'lay' perspective, as 'experts by experience' or more generally as recipients of services. To highlight the importance of engaging with service users and carers, additional information is included in section 3.4 regarding their involvement.

It is therefore essential that all potential stakeholders, who may have an interest in a specific guideline topic, are identified at the initial planning stage of the project. When a topic is being considered for a guideline project, relevant stakeholder organisations should be invited to register their interest and, where indicated, discuss their potential involvement in guideline development activities.

It is unlikely that all potential stakeholders will be able or wish to be involved either in the guideline development group or at all stages of the guideline development process. Occupational therapy is delivered in a wide range of services and environments and, therefore, the most appropriate approach to involvement of any individual stakeholder will be influenced by service delivery configurations, professional networks, and the knowledge and experience of individuals and organisations in the topic field.

Key points: Stakeholder involvement

The following should be considered:

- Who are the key stakeholders who should be invited to be members of the guideline development group or a reference group? The aim should be to include the most appropriate stakeholder representatives on the core guideline development group, which will normally consist of up to eight members.

- What is the relationship between each potential stakeholder and service users, carers or the occupational therapy service in question?

- What level of involvement will each identified stakeholder have? For example, contributing to the scoping process; full member of the guideline development group; co-opted expert opinion at specific stages; reviewing document drafts; external peer review; providing a foreword; or co-badging a publication.

- Expectations of involvement should be discussed and agreed with the invited stakeholders before the process begins.

- The project lead should explain the College's policy for expenses for lay people (lay representatives and service users/carers).

- Identified key stakeholders must have the opportunity to influence the development of the scope (that is, what is to be included and excluded within the guideline).

- Identified key stakeholders must be consulted on an early draft of a guideline document and/or a quick reference guide version.

- Stakeholders should be officially contacted by the project lead or a member of the College's Specialist Section (where leading the guideline development).

Potential stakeholders will most probably be known to the project lead and Specialist Section members, but additional organisations may be identified by looking at stakeholder lists used by the National Institute for Health and Care Excellence (*http://www.nice.org.uk/guidance*) and the Scottish Intercollegiate Guidelines Network (SIGN) (*http://www.sign.ac.uk/patients/resources.html*).

There is no one single model of stakeholder involvement that will suit all guideline development projects, so it is important that the project lead is able to rationalise, evidence and document their approach to engagement.

3.4 Service user and carer involvement

Service users and carers are important stakeholders. Individuals and/or groups should be invited to be part of guideline development. Opportunities and options for engaging service users and/or carers in the specific guideline project will need to be identified at the initial planning stage of the project.

Once identified, access to service users and carers may depend to some extent on the networks that the guideline development group members already have established or of which they are aware.

Occupational therapists work across a wide range of specialties. They may work with individuals who have particular needs with respect to communication or mental capacity, and therefore their engagement in the guideline development process may have additional requirements.

Key points: Service user and carer involvement

The following should be considered:

- Time may be required to ensure that service users and carers are fully informed about the role of occupational therapy, the nature of practice guidelines and the expectations and boundaries of involvement.

- Information to share with service users about getting involved in guideline development should be provided, with the opportunity to discuss the content further with a member of the guideline development group or an officer of the College of Occupational Therapists.

- The level of involvement may vary for different service users/carers: for example, contributing to the scoping process; full member of the guideline development group (potentially as a representative of a formal lay or service user organisation); co-opted 'lived experience' expert opinion at specific stages; reviewing document drafts; or providing a foreword. This should be discussed and agreed with the invited service user(s)/carer(s).

- Where appropriate forums exist for service users or carers, with established contact systems and opportunities for engagement (for example, via charitable organisation member forums), then these may provide both a realistic and practical option for involvement.

- The needs of the specific guideline population will mean that different approaches may be required to maximise involvement of the service user/carer representatives. This could include, for example, membership of the core guideline development group or a reference/advisory group; attendance at individual meetings or focus groups; or participation via telephone or email.

- Where indicated, creative approaches may be required to engage those with more complex needs, and to ensure that information is fully accessible (for example, talking mats, visual analogue scales) and does not create a barrier to inclusion.

- The support that may be required for an individual to contribute effectively to a formal guideline development group meeting should not be underestimated.

- The project lead should explain the College's policy for expenses for lay people (lay representatives and service users/carers).

- Service user and carer representatives must have the opportunity to influence the development of the scope.

- Service user and carer representatives must be consulted on an early draft document.

- Service user and carer representatives should be officially contacted by the Project Lead or another member of the project group).

- There is no one single model of service user/carer involvement that will suit all guideline development projects, so it is important that the project lead is able to rationalise and evidence their approach to engagement.

Evidence, relevant to the guideline scope, which uses a qualitative methodology to investigate service user and carer perspectives, will automatically be included in a guideline topic literature search and considered in the subsequent stages of the guideline development process.

Any specific involvement of service users or carers outside of 'consultation' may potentially be deemed as research, and therefore consideration must be given as to whether research ethics approval is required. Research in this context should be seen as a separate project to the guideline development. Advice should be sought from the College's Education and Research Team regarding potential research governance requirements.

3.5 Scope and purpose of the guideline

The first key task for the guideline development group is to discuss and agree the scope of the proposed guideline. The resulting document or 'scope' will become the framework for the guideline. It therefore needs to be well-considered and clearly defined (see Appendices 2 and 3).

The scope sets the parameters and describes what is to be included and excluded and should be agreed by consultation with relevant stakeholders. The scope should include consideration of potential health inequalities, and any social determinants of health, that may be appropriate to the guideline, i.e. best start in life for children; fair employment and good work for all; healthy standard of living for all; maximising individual capability and control over life; creating and developing healthy and sustainable places and communities; and strengthening the role and impact of ill-health prevention (Marmot 2010, p15).

Key points: The scope

This needs to specify areas including:

- The provisional guideline title.

- The overall objective of the guideline.

- The background:

  - current role and relevance of occupational therapy

  - the need for the guideline

  - who may be interested in the guideline

- an explanation of the condition/situation
- the frequency of the condition/situation.
- Practice questions to be addressed by the guideline.
- The population:
  - age group to be covered
  - gender issues where appropriate
  - ethnic or cultural considerations where appropriate
  - potential health inequalities
  - particular sub-groups that will not be covered, with rationale for exclusion.
- The setting, i.e. the specific clinical, healthcare, social or other circumstances.
- How the guideline content will support an occupation-centred focus to practice.
- Key outcomes anticipated for service users.
- The areas of intervention/action to be covered and any comparisons.
- The areas of intervention/action that will not be covered, with rationale for exclusion.
- Anticipated impact of an occupational therapy practice guideline on this topic.
- The possible range of tools to support implementation.
- The target audience.

3.6 Developing the clinical, healthcare or social practice questions

The recommendations in a guideline should provide a response to specific clinical, healthcare or social practice question(s). Specificity is important in developing questions which address the requirements of the scope, and to subsequently ensure that the appropriate evidence can be identified and retrieved within the search.

Key points: The PICO methodology

Questions should contain four key elements:

- The **P**atient (service user), **P**opulation or **P**roblem/circumstance.
- The **I**ntervention under investigation or action.
- The **C**omparison, which is an alternative intervention or action.
- The desired **O**utcome.

(Richardson et al 1995)

The patient (service user), population or problem/circumstance defines the care group or condition that is being studied, or it may be a specific functional/occupational need. This group or situation needs to be defined in detail and include, for example, age, gender and location.

The intervention defines an intervention or action that would be used for this group or situation. The comparison (or alternative intervention) describes another possible action or approach that could be taken and may be used within the question as a comparison. In occupational therapy there may not be an alternative intervention or action, in which case it need not be included.

The outcome should describe the desired/undesired or expected result of the intervention. It is important to highlight and consider the significance of the outcomes to the service user and the potential improvement to their occupational performance.

3.7 Finding the supporting knowledge and evidence

Developing an evidence-based guideline requires a systematic approach to the search and the review of the literature. Woolf et al (2012) suggest that this is a critical stage of guideline development which should include defining which types of evidence and information will be relevant, and by what criteria that evidence will be evaluated.

What is meant by 'best evidence' can be a matter of some debate. Evidence-based practice has its origins in medicine, but it has evolved as a concept which fully recognises that it is not 'just research' (Sackett et al 2000). It takes into account the integration of the best available research evidence, together with the practitioner's clinical expertise and the service user's values and goals.

The Social Care Institute of Excellence (SCIE) acknowledges that a rigid, research-based notion of evidence does not fit easily with the social care evidence base, and has introduced a broader concept of 'knowledge'. This encompasses a variety of methodological traditions as well as the everyday expertise and experience of stakeholders, including service users. SCIE does not identify a specific hierarchy of evidence, preferring to highlight the source of the evidence and indicating that all sources have a role to play in building up the social care evidence base (Pawson et al 2003).

Key points: SCIE classification of knowledge

- Organisational knowledge: information, regulations and requirements generated by an organisation to govern its activity – often incorporated in the background section of a guideline.

- Practitioner knowledge: an individual's knowledge acquired through practice, education, advice and liaison – usually involved as part of guideline development group or peer review.

- User knowledge: information generated by users and carers from their experience – usually gained via involvement in the guideline development group or its activities and possibly in evidence identified.

- Research knowledge: knowledge generated through formal research methods – identified from searching for research studies.

- Policy community knowledge: broad principles, strategies and information concerning social care within the political, social and economic environment – often incorporated in the background section of a guideline.

(based on Pawson et al 2003)

Much of occupational therapy is about enabling an individual to access 'occupation' in its broadest terms. It may only be possible to measure such activity and the outcomes for the individual in descriptive and qualitative terms and therefore the sources of information and evidence accessed should be as inclusive as possible, and take into consideration the framework of sources, as outlined by SCIE.

Sources of evidence will extend beyond electronically held information, and there is potentially invaluable grey literature that may need to be accessed by handsearching.

Key points: Types of evidence

The range of knowledge or evidence to be appraised may include:

- Systematic reviews.

- Randomised controlled trials (RCTs).

- Non-randomised experimental research single study designs.

- Surveys.

- Qualitative research studies.

- Cost effectiveness/economic evaluation studies.

- Opinion pieces.

- Policy experience.

- Service evaluations.

- Expert opinion based on consensus (for example, Delphi survey findings).

- Service user information.

- Other grey literature (for example, unpublished documents, theses, government reports).

In order to inform the search, it is necessary to be very clear about what is required and the keywords that best reflect the questions to be answered, thus defining the nature and scope of the search carefully. This should be sufficiently comprehensive to give a balance of high sensitivity (the number of studies located on the topic) and also provide high specificity (the number of relevant studies, i.e. the ratio between the 'hits' and 'misses'). If not, the evidence that is found may be incomplete, potentially giving an inaccurate bias to the finished guideline.

The College of Occupational Therapists Library and Information Service undertakes literature searches for practice guideline development using core databases:

- EBSCOhost platform: CINAHL, MEDLINE.

- OVID platform: Allied and Complementary Medicine (AMED), PsycINFO, Social Policy and Practice, and Health Management Information Consortium (HMIC).

The librarians will select other databases as appropriate to the guideline topic. Other specialist databases which can be accessed are OTDBASE, OT SEARCH, OTseeker, Cochrane Library, NICE and SIGN guidelines and the College's own specialist occupational therapy literature catalogue.

> **Key points: The search strategy**
>
> This should identify:
>
> - The exact search terms and the rationale for their use (with reference to international descriptions of conditions, service user groups and spelling variations).
>
> - Key occupation-focused terminology/language.
>
> - Any language restrictions.
>
> - The relevant setting (for example, hospitals, schools, workplaces, in the community or other environments where occupational therapy is provided).
>
> - Whether the search is limited to the United Kingdom or wider.
>
> - How recent the evidence needs to be, with time period specified.
>
> - The most appropriate sources and the specific databases used, which will depend upon the nature of the material required.

The search strategy and process must be recorded to a level of detail that would enable it to be subsequently re-run. This means that another group could repeat the process by the same method and should reach the same conclusions. The strategy, search terms (including Boolean operators and database syntaxes), date and outcomes of the search must be made explicit in the guideline document to avoid any misinterpretation. The full search history and results should be available on request.

3.8 Appraising the evidence

Specific inclusion and exclusion criteria must be developed prior to screening the results of the literature search. These criteria must be specified and justified within the guideline document. The search results will need to be screened and reviewed against the defined criteria to enable the most appropriate sources of evidence to be appraised. It may be possible to identify the appropriate evidence to be included from the abstracts, but where there is uncertainty, the full paper will be required. It is not advisable that decisions at any stage of the screening or appraisal process be made by only one person, as this opens up the possibility of human error or bias.

Articles excluded from critical appraisal, particularly those that just fall short of inclusion criteria and that the reader may expect to see included, should be recorded with a brief reason. This may be documented within the main text or as an appendix if there are a large number of excluded papers.

The strengths and limitations of the body of evidence should be highlighted and any areas of uncertainty acknowledged.

Having identified and located the knowledge or evidence that might be suitable or useful, each piece of included evidence needs to be critically appraised to decide whether it is good quality and whether it is appropriate for the guideline purpose.

Key points: Appraising the evidence

General principles to consider when reviewing the value of any evidence:

• The evidence must be of relevance to both the practitioners and the service users in the field of practice under consideration, in order to assist in the decision-making process.

• The evidence should be as recent as possible. It will no longer be of relevance if practice has significantly developed subsequent to the publication of that evidence.

• The evidence should enable the guideline development group to take account of the clinical or practical effectiveness of any interventions or actions. The guideline development group will need to be able to assess both the benefits and the risks of any actions or interventions.

• The guideline development group should consider evidence of the cost effectiveness of any interventions or actions. This may include a cost/benefit analysis and/or comparison to other interventions. This could present a challenge unless a member of the group has a health economics background.

• The guideline development group should consider evidence that reflects service users' experiences and preferences and include these as appropriate within the guideline.

The process of appraisal aims to assess the methodological rigour and potential bias of any evidence. Because different types of research have specific interpretations of rigour, based on particular methodological perspectives, it is important that the correct criteria and appraisal tools are used for the various types of research.

Appraising the evidence can be a time-consuming task. It is important to have one or more guideline development group members who have a breadth of research knowledge and who are skilled and experienced in the critical appraisal of evidence. A minimum of two guideline development group members should carry out an independent appraisal of each included article. In the case of appraisal by only two members, any differences in assessment or assignment of level of quality should be discussed between the two appraisers and, if necessary, with a third person or the full guideline development group to reach an agreed decision.

A rigorous methodology is required and the College, whilst recognising there are a variety of appraisal tools available, requires that either the McMaster University Critical Review Forms or the Critical Appraisal Skills Programme (CASP) tools are used as standard. Both these resources provide frameworks that can be used to appraise different types of studies. They can be accessed, subject to copyright requirements, via the McMaster University or CASP UK websites respectively (Appendix 4). Details of the tool(s) used must be recorded in the guidelines.

A flowchart should be produced to clarify the number of articles identified, and decisions made regarding inclusion/exclusion, at each stage of the article search, selection and appraisal process.

Evidence tables should be used for summarising information and recording decisions made about each study appraised. It is recommended that these tables are included as an appendix in guideline products (Appendix 5).

3.9 Grading quality of evidence – GRADE

A number of grading systems exist for deciding on the quality of the available evidence. The College has adopted elements of the GRADE system (Grading of Recommendations Assessment, Development and Evaluation, *http://www.gradeworkinggroup.org/*) for evaluation of quality of evidence and the subsequent decision about the strength of a guideline recommendation.

GRADE, developed by a widely representative group of international guideline developers, is being used by a number of organisations and provides measures for both quality of evidence and strength of recommendations. The grading system enables guidelines to be developed that are not dependent on the availability of randomised controlled trials and takes into account factors influencing the quality and limitations of studies.

Quality of evidence reflects the extent to which there can be confidence in the 'estimate of the effect' or the outcome described by the research, and although 'quality' should be seen as a continuum, categorisation offers 'simplicity and transparency' (Guyatt et al 2008a).

The design of a study provides the underpinning framework for determining quality, acknowledging that, in general, stronger evidence is provided by randomised controlled trials (RCTs) compared to observational studies, and that rigorous observational studies provide stronger evidence than uncontrolled case series. Expert opinion is included in this grading system and the College interprets this as inclusive of the service user experience.

Under the GRADE categorisation, where there are no important limitations, RCTs constitute high-quality evidence, and observational studies without special strengths or important limitations constitute low-quality evidence. All other evidence constitutes very low-quality evidence (GRADE Working Group 2004).

This type of grading system, like a number of others, has a stronger association with medical research, where more frequently there is the availability of evidence from large scale randomised controlled trials. The nature of occupational therapy research is much broader, and there is, in particular, an important body of high-quality qualitative research. It is imperative to recognise, therefore, that the grading allocated for occupational therapy evidence may in many cases be low or very low. The College's view, however, is that this does not negate the potential significance of such research, and its important contribution to practice guideline recommendations. This may be reflected in a recommendation, based on qualitative evidence, being categorised as strong rather than conditional.

Following appraisal, quality of the available evidence for a given outcome should be given an initial grading in one of the following categories:

• Randomised trial/systematic review = high

• Observational study = low

• Any other evidence = very low.

Limitations in the design of a study and its implementation may, however, bias the estimates of the treatment effect. If there are serious limitations, then downgrading of the quality of the evidence should be considered by the guideline development group.

Table 1 Upgrading and downgrading quality

Decrease* grade if	• Serious or very serious limitation to study quality. • Important inconsistencies in results. • Some or major uncertainty about directness of the evidence. • Imprecise or sparse data (relatively few participants and/or events). • High probability of reporting bias.
Increase grade if	• Magnitude of the treatment effect is very large and consistent. • Evidence of a large dose–response relationship. • All plausible confounders/biases would have decreased the magnitude of an apparent treatment effect. *Only studies with no major threats to validity should be upgraded.*

* Each quality criterion can reduce the quality by one or, if very serious, by two levels.

(based on GRADE Working Group 2004)

Decisions in relation to up or downgrading evidence require judgement should be explicit and transparent.

Depending on the various factors detailed in Table 1, the initial grading may potentially be increased or decreased. Evidence will ultimately be finally graded in one of four categories from high to very low, as defined in Table 2. To facilitate ease of identification, the College uses an alphabetical reference for this grading from A (high) to D (very low).

Table 2 GRADE quality of evidence grading

Quality of evidence	The College's grading for quality of evidence	Characteristics	Confidence
High	Grade A	Based on consistent results from well-performed randomised controlled trials, or overwhelming evidence of an alternative source e.g. well-executed observational studies with strong effects.	True effect lies close to that of the estimate of the effect. Further research is very unlikely to change confidence in the estimate of the effect.
Moderate	Grade B	Based on randomised controlled trials where there are serious flaws in conduct, inconsistency, indirectness, imprecise estimates, reporting bias or some other combination of these limitations, or from other study designs with special strengths.	True effect likely to be close to the estimate of the effect, but there is a possibility that there could be a substantial difference. Further research is likely to have an important impact on our confidence in the estimate of effect and may change the estimate.

Low	Grade C	Based on observational evidence, or from controlled trials with several very serious limitations.	True effect may be substantially different from the estimate of the effect. Further research is very likely to have an important impact on confidence in the estimate of the effect and is likely to change the estimate.
Very Low	Grade D	Based on case studies or expert opinion.	Any estimate of effect is very uncertain and may be far from the true effect.

3.10 Formulating and grading recommendations

Guidelines inform decision-making and make recommendations about the actions that should be taken in a given situation or for the population concerned. The literature search will have identified material evidence or expert opinions in response to the original guideline questions. The review and evaluation will have identified the highest-quality evidence or knowledge that gives the clearest guidance as to what is best practice.

Once the methodological quality of each piece of evidence has been assessed, it can then be evaluated to judge its potential contribution to the development of the guideline recommendations. The best available evidence identified should be synthesised and used to formulate the recommendations.

Evidence may not necessarily be explicit or unambiguous with respect to formulating the recommendations. Where a number of items of evidence are supporting an identified outcome and subsequent recommendation, an overall quality of evidence rating should be identified:

- If the evidence outcomes point in different directions towards benefit and towards harm, the lowest quality of evidence should determine the overall quality of evidence.

- If the outcomes point in the same direction towards either benefit or harm, then the highest quality of evidence should be appropriate to recommend an intervention and will determine the overall quality of evidence.

- In circumstances where the balance of benefits and harm is uncertain, then the lowest grade of quality of evidence should be assigned.

GRADE highlights that not all high-quality evidence results in an automatically strong recommendation, and vice versa.

Risks: any recommendation that has an element of risk within it should be assessed in the light of whether there is a need for some positive risk within the occupational therapy process. Risk management considerations may then form part of the recommendation.

Key points: Defining a recommendation

The guideline development group should consider a number of factors:

- Rating of methodological quality of the evidence.

- Uncertainty in the estimates of likely benefit/risk.

- Importance of the outcome.

- Quantity, strength, quality and consistency of evidence.

- Whether the findings of the study can be generalised.

- Applicability to the target population of the guideline.

- Impact on service users (that is, the extent of the impact on the target population).

- Risks and benefits associated with the intervention, including any side-effects/contra-indications.

- Resources needed to implement the recommendations into the workplace.

Barriers to implementation: it is also essential that any potential organisational, resourcing or financial barriers that may exist, which could affect implementation (National Institute for Health and Care Excellence 2015), are discussed and documented.

Key points: Recommendation statements

Recommendations should:

- Be objective, clear and unambiguous and precise in describing the desired activity/procedure.

- Not incorporate personal or subjective opinion and should be transparent about, and take account of, any potential for bias.

- State the specific clinical, healthcare, social or other circumstances.

- Clearly present different options for the management of the condition or options for intervention, where appropriate.

- Be supported and referenced to the evidence or knowledge used in their development.

- Identify specifically if they are based on expert opinion/consensus.

- Make explicit the links between the recommendation and the evidence on which it is based.

In developing the recommendations, any limitations within the guideline development process should be explained and documented: for example, a poor response from identified stakeholders, or limitations of search or evidence findings (which may include applicability for culture or context).

3.11 Strength and overall grading of recommendations

Strength of recommendation is the second element of the GRADE system and the College uses the following two categories, strong or conditional, to reflect the strength. Assigning a recommendation as either strong or conditional provides the guideline user with a clear indication of the level of confidence.

Key points: Factors affecting strength of a recommendation

The strength of a recommendation will be influenced by a number of determinants (Guyatt et al 2008b) but in particular reflects:

- The extent of confidence that the benefits or desirable effects of the intervention outweigh the risks or undesirable effects, or vice versa, across the range of individuals for whom the recommendation is intended.

- That the quality of the evidence as a strong recommendation requires certainty about the magnitude of benefits and harm of an intervention.

- Uncertainty about, or variability in, values and preferences about this intervention compared to alternatives (view of guideline development group).

- Resources/costs required.

The strength of grade assigned will also reflect the characteristics below in Table 3.

Table 3 Strength of grade

Strength	Grade	Benefits and risks	Implications
Strong	1 'It is recommended . . .'	Benefits appear to outweigh the risks (or vice versa) for the majority of the target group.	Most service users would want to, or should, receive this course of intervention or action.
Conditional	2 'It is suggested . . .'	Risks and benefits are more closely balanced, or there is more uncertainty in likely service user values and preferences.	The majority of service users would want this intervention, but not all, and, therefore, they should be supported to arrive at a decision for intervention consistent with the benefits, and their values and preferences.

(based on Guyatt et al 2008b)

A recommendation decision form should be completed for each recommendation developed, recording key information about the evidence used to form the basis of that recommendation, and the overall allocation of quality of evidence and strength of recommendation. Any judgement by the guideline development group should be documented as part of this decision-making process (see section 3.17 and Appendix 6). The information recorded should be summarised within the main guideline text to ensure there is a clear association and logical development from the appraisal of the evidence and the recommendation.

Key points: Overall grade of a recommendation

The overall grade of a recommendation is depicted in a guideline document with a numerical, then alphabetical, grade to reflect the strength and quality of evidence e.g. 1A – Strong, high-quality; 2C – Conditional, low-quality.

3.12 Writing the guideline

The editorial role is important to ensure that the guideline meets all the College's requirements relating to content, style and format, and to ensure that the language is clear, specific and unambiguous. As such, a designated editorial lead is required. This role can be undertaken by either a member of the guideline development group or by the College. In both cases any potential conflict of interest must be declared and recorded. Editorial support provided by the College does not include determining the nature and content of the recommendations. These decisions are the responsibility of the guideline development group.

Key points: Clarity and presentation of the guideline

- Guideline products should be tailored to meet the needs of the primary audience and, where appropriate, alternative formats should be made available (for example, for service users).

- Attention should be given to the language used to write the guideline, ensuring it is professional and appropriate to the target audience(s):

  - Stick to a jargon-free, plain English style – write concisely and clearly.

  - Use the active rather than passive voice where possible.

  - Use positive presentations of ethnicity, gender, age and physical characteristics.

  - Ensure that all definitions and terminology used are current.

- To facilitate ease of use, recommendation statements need to be instantly recognisable from the main body of text, and a quick reference summary should be provided at the front of the document.

- Guidelines should be structured in a logical and methodical way, ensuring that all stages of the process are documented accurately (Appendix 7).

- Where appropriate, a guideline should be linked to other professional documents. It is better to reference a section of another document than to repeat it at length.

Future research: where gaps in the evidence or research priorities are identified, these can inform the future research agenda and should be detailed in the guideline document.

3.13 Peer review

Peer review may be provided by a number of different individuals or groups. It is important to assess a number of factors, including content, validity, reliability and potential applicability/usefulness in practice.

> **Key points: Peer review**
>
> The College peer review process includes:
>
> - The College Practice Publications Group provides a specific peer review process with reference to the scoping proposal and draft guideline document meeting key criteria (see section 5.1).
>
> - Specialist Section(s) involved in leading a guideline development project are required to seek peer review on the draft guideline document via open consultation with their members/occupational therapists, who are the largest potential group of end users of the document. A stakeholder feedback form will be provided.
>
> - Independent experts (a minimum of two) will be officially invited by the project lead to provide a peer review. These individuals should have the relevant experience and be acknowledged experts in the topic and/or in guideline development. Responses should be provided in a standard format (Appendix 8) to the project and editorial leads.
>
> - A period of one month should be allowed for peer review responses.
>
> - All peer reviewers must be asked to declare any conflict of interest.

Peer review essentially represents a 'field test', and should be carried out using a high-quality and complete agreed full draft of the guideline document. The guideline development group will need to factor in the time for review of feedback and the incorporation of amendments.

3.14 Review and updating

Published guidelines must be reviewed after a certain time. An alert system should be in place to highlight new evidence pertinent to the guideline scope post-publication. This is crucial to ensure that the recommendations remain applicable, accurate and up to date. The College recommends formal review commences at a maximum period of three to five years from publication or the previous review. This period should be reduced if significant new evidence becomes available that would alter the recommendations, to ensure quality and relevance of the guideline is maintained.

The College keeps an overview of all published guidelines and the scheduled review dates. The original developers or initiators of the guideline are responsible for implementing its review. This should be done by a group of experts similar to the original guideline development group, although it does not have to be the same people.

The review needs to ascertain whether there is suitable new knowledge or evidence. If so, this would need to be appraised. Any original material that is no longer appropriate, for example out of date or superseded, should be withdrawn. The recommendations should also be updated if indicated by new evidence or knowledge. New recommendations should be identified in the revised document.

If the use of the original guideline has initiated useful feedback and comments, these can be incorporated into a revision if agreed by the review group.

The review and updating procedure must be thorough and should follow the details found in section 5.7.

3.15 Funding mechanisms for guideline development

As a membership organisation, the major source of funding for the College of Occupational Therapists is obtained from its membership. Other sources of income are primarily from advertising and events. A copy of the College's statutory accounts is available from its website (*https://www.cot.co.uk/annual-reviews/annual-reviews*).

Occupational therapy practice guidelines are commonly developed by a group led by a Specialist Section of the College. These are official branches of the College who, through their membership, are able to engage expert practitioners, educators and researchers in the development of guidelines, and access the required clinical and research expertise. Further information about Specialist Sections can be accessed from the College's website.

If the project is being led by a College Specialist Section, then it must have the written support of the section Chair. The proposed publication should be discussed with the executive committee and their networks should be utilised to recruit group members with specific skills as required. Discussions with the committee should also result in an agreement of funding that will be ring-fenced within their budget to support the development of the guideline. It is important that the amount of funding is established at an early stage, as this will influence the scope of what the group can undertake and achieve. It can also help the group to decide whether additional funding needs to be sought from elsewhere.

Specific costs may also be met by the College. These are limited to travel expenses to attend meetings, photocopying and publishing costs.

All funding sources must be declared in the published guideline document.

3.16 Conflicts of interest

All individuals and organisations involved in developing practice guidelines must declare any conflicts of interest in relation to their intended or ongoing involvement in the guideline development process and associated activities. This statement is in line with the College of Occupational Therapists' *Policy on conflicts of interest* (COT 2015a).

Key points: Conflict of interest

This is identified as either a personal (of the person, their partner or close relatives) or a non-personal (of their department/employer/business) interest, which could have the potential to influence or affect their contribution to the development or content of occupational therapy guidelines. Interests may be financial or non-financial, or commercial. Interests can be considered as either 'specific' to the guideline topic or meeting agenda (e.g. authorship of evidence being considered) or 'non-specific' (e.g. member of a Specialist Section or professional body).

The nature of the activities and expertise of those involved in the development of occupational therapy guidelines mean that a conflict of interest may potentially occur. It is important that any relevant or associated issues, even though they may not be directly considered a conflict of interest, are highlighted, discussed and recorded. This applies to members of the guideline development group and all others who contribute to any specific elements/stages of the process: for example, external peer reviewers. Any change in interests during the course of the individual's involvement in the guideline development must also be notified and recorded.

A conflicts of interest declaration form (Appendix 9) must be completed by all involved and will be held by the project lead until the guideline is completed. Subsequent forms will be stored by the College in line with data retention guidance.

Dependent on the type of conflict, an individual may not be able to contribute to the guideline development process in whole or part. Appendix 10 provides detailed information on managing conflicts of interest within an occupational therapy guideline development group.

3.17 Decision-making processes

The guideline development group should adopt a consensus approach to decision-making. This involves participation and open discussion by **all** members, which should result in a decision that the group as a whole is able to support. The recommendation statements, for example, including assignment of the overall quality and strength grading, should be agreed using this decision-making process.

If a decision cannot be reached by consensus the Chair will need to ask all members in attendance at the meeting to take a vote. Where a majority vote is not reached, the Chair or Vice-Chair (depending on any declared conflicts of interest) will have the deciding vote.

The method used to obtain agreement must be described in the guideline document, with the outcome of any voting decisions recorded in the meeting minutes.

4 Implementation of guidelines

The purpose of a practice guideline is to bring about positive change, both in the quality and consistency of practice and in the outcomes and experiences for service users. The publication of the guideline document in itself will not bring about the desired change. It has to become part of everyday practice. Awareness and knowledge of what needs to change, and why, are vital first steps in enabling change to occur (NICE 2007).

The implementation of any guideline needs to be an active process. Multiple approaches are likely to be more effective than a single one. Implementation can benefit from having influential people sponsoring or supporting the document. However, the ongoing use of a guideline will be determined by the degree to which it actually assists commissioners and practitioners in decision-making and problem-solving. Guidelines must be 'owned' by practitioners across whole systems of care or the service. In this way equity and continuity of service provision can develop.

Implementation strategies to support guideline uptake are important. Shekelle et al (2012) suggest that implementability can be enhanced by the relationship with those responsible for dissemination and implementation. The College works with its Specialist Sections to incorporate strategies such as multiple formats and channels for dissemination; development of educational resources; and use of data collection tools (such as simple audit templates).

4.1 Selecting implementation techniques and support tools

Implementation will need to take place at a local level, taking into account circumstances and systems in that setting, including identification and discussion of the potential organisational and financial barriers to implementation detailed in the guideline document.

Occupational therapists working in the guideline area of practice will need, both individually and as a service, to review the guideline as part of their evidence-based practice activities, in line with the requirements of the Health and Care Professions Council (HCPC 2013) and the College's *Code of ethics and professional conduct* (COT 2015b). Bringing the guideline to the attention of the relevant clinical governance/audit or equivalent department is also recommended, particularly as they may have established mechanisms or strategies for implementation, and be able to provide support and audit. A guideline should also be brought to the attention of managers and commissioners.

The guideline development group should give consideration to how the guideline may be implemented by practitioners, and develop support tools to facilitate its use.

The College of Occupational Therapists will coordinate the production of a core set of implementation resources for each guideline. These aim to facilitate an implementation pathway of awareness, audit and application of a new guideline, and will be made available to download from the College website.

Guideline development groups will be encouraged to submit abstracts for professional conferences and articles within relevant publications.

Key points: Support tools

The core set of implementation resources produced for each guideline include:

- Continuing professional development/knowledge transfer resource: an interactive resource that can be tailored for local use. The session can be used for group or self-directed learning, or for raising awareness of the guideline at multidisciplinary meetings and study days/events.

- Quick reference guide, which provides the recommendations and key information in a concise, easy-to-use format for practitioners.

- Audit support form with defined criteria and data collection guidance.

- Implementation tips: practical tips to support the translation of recommendations into practice.

Additional resources that can be considered include:

- Costing tools to estimate the financial aspects of implementation, including running costs and potential long-term savings.

- Fact sheets for managers/commissioners.

- Service user information to raise awareness of an occupational therapist's role in a particular area of practice.

5 The College's appraisal and approval process

5.1 Practice Publications Group

In order to provide accurate and timely information for occupational therapists nationally, the College has established a clear and rigorous publication process. The College's Practice Publications Group (PPG) oversees the process and provides a quality assurance role. It reviews guideline proposals and drafts produced by members who wish to publish in collaboration with the College.

The terms of reference for the PPG are available in Appendix 11 and outline membership of the group.

5.2 Guideline appraisal

Practice guidelines are assessed by the PPG against the *Appraisal of guidelines, research and evaluation (AGREE) II instrument* (AGREE Next Steps Consortium 2013), which was developed by an international collaboration of researchers and policy-makers. It aims to improve the quality and effectiveness of clinical practice guidelines by establishing a shared framework for their development, reporting and assessment. The instrument is designed to assess guidelines developed at all levels, from local to international groups.

The *AGREE II instrument* provides a framework for this assessment against six different aspects or domains: scope and purpose; stakeholder involvement; rigour of development; clarity and presentation; applicability; and editorial independence. The instrument is available with guidance to download. These domains and their associated criteria are also compatible with the NICE Accreditation scheme requirements (National Institute for Health and Care Excellence 2014).

Provided that the guideline has followed the College's development process and that the recommendations reflect the status of the evidence base, this assessment is used to enable the PPG to make a final decision regarding the approval and ratification of a guideline document.

5.3 Guideline development timeline

The practice guideline development process has been set out in three stages, with a total of eighteen steps, to ensure that guidelines are developed using a rigorous and robust methodology and a process that aims to meet national quality standards.

The College fully recognises that most members of the occupational therapy profession contributing to guideline development will be undertaking a significant proportion (if not all) of the activities required within their personal time, and will not always receive paid leave to facilitate attendance at meetings. The project lead will, therefore, need to facilitate a balance between maintaining momentum and progress of the project, and the needs of the guideline development group. This should be considered when drawing up a project plan to ensure the timescales are achievable.

A guideline development group is expected to complete its project in 18–24 months, with the three stages broken down into the following anticipated timescales:

Proposal stage	3–5 months
Development stage	11–13 months
Approval and publication stage	3–4 months

It is recognised, however, that at each stage targets may be influenced by factors such as the volume of evidence, and the existing commitments of group members and those who are contacted for expert advice and contributions.

Following publication of the guideline, the process for review and updating needs to be followed as outlined in section 5.7.

5.4 Proposal stage (3–5 months)

i. Potential guideline topic identified by Specialist Section/other group (see also 3.1)
Specialist Sections or other groups identifying a need for a practice guideline for occupational therapy should in the first instance contact the College's Quality Programme Manager to discuss the potential need or demand for the practice guideline and the likelihood of support from the College. The College is not in a position to support all requests and groups should consider the questions highlighted in 'selecting a topic' (see section 3.1) before planning a guideline project.

ii. Advisory meeting (see also 3.3, 3.4, 3.15)
Where proposals for potential guidelines may be viable to progress, the guideline proposer will be invited to attend an advisory meeting at the College. The proposer should be familiar with the content and requirements of this manual prior to the meeting.

This meeting aims to explore the provisional idea further, and to explain key requirements and stages of the development process. This will include discussion of:

• Guideline development group membership and skills.

• Service user/carer and stakeholder involvement expectations.

• Support available from the College.

• The ongoing commitment required from a Specialist Section to support the development, post-publication evaluation, review and updating of a guideline.

• Funding requirements.

• The timeline and milestones for the development period.

iii. Proposal submitted to the PPG (see also 3.2)
The proposal form can be obtained by emailing the College's Quality Programme Manager (a copy of this can also be found in Appendix 1).

When submitting the form, the project lead must provide written confirmation from the Chair of the Specialist Section or group, confirming the committee's support and designated funding. The proposal should include details of the stakeholders contacted and the expressions of interest received to support the development of the guideline. The completed form should be returned to the College's Quality Programme Manager so that it can be considered by the PPG.

Proposals which have been approved by the PPG and College will be recommended to proceed to the scoping stage and the project lead will be sent information regarding copyright assignment.

iv. Scope and project plan developed by the guideline development group (see also 3.5, 3.6, 3.16)

The project lead will need to convene a meeting of the guideline development group.

Discussions should focus on:

- Clarifying the future roles and responsibilities of the group members.

- The involvement and engagement of all stakeholders.

- Developing the draft scope.

- Arrangements for the consultation of the draft scope with stakeholders.

- The process for revising the scope following consultation.

- The timescales and agreed milestones for the project.

The draft scope should be sent to stakeholders for comment (see Appendix 3) to ensure that all views are represented in the final version.

v. Submit guideline development project scope to the PPG

The next stage of the process involves submitting a scope form, an example of which is provided in Appendix 2, and the detailed project plan/chart (action plan) to the PPG for review.

A copy of the final scope, together with stakeholder comments and the guideline development group's responses, should also be provided.

Once the PPG has approved the scope, the project can progress to the development stage.

PROPOSAL STAGE FLOWCHART

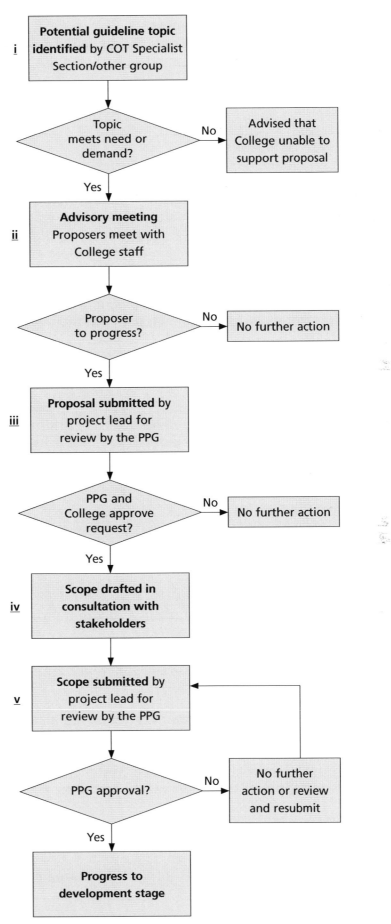

5.5 Development stage (11–13 months)

vi. Guideline development commences
Provided that the PPG approves the scope, the guideline development group can proceed with the development of the guideline. Once this stage has been reached, a number of College resources will be available to the group. Appendix 12 outlines these resources and Appendix 13 explains the guideline development group's responsibilities.

vii. Literature search (see also 3.7)
The search terms included on the scope form will be used to inform the search strategy developed by the College's Library. The search strategy will be the focus of the next guideline development group meeting which will be attended by College librarians. Once the strategy is agreed the final database searching will be undertaken and results provided via the Project Lead.

Group members are asked to note that this search is not exhaustive and that they will also be expected to conduct additional literature searching (for example, handsearching of relevant reference lists). Guideline development groups are also advised that it may be easier, in some instances, to source material from their own host organisation libraries.

At this stage the Editorial Lead must ensure that all necessary details of the search are recorded.

viii. Guideline development group review search findings
The development of inclusion and exclusion criteria for evidence should be completed prior to review of the search findings. Those criteria will be used to direct the screening of the search results and the decisions on those articles to be sourced for appraisal.

ix. Critical appraisal (see also 3.8, 3.9)
Critical appraisal will need to be carried out by at least two members of the group to provide an independent review of each article or literature source. A research and development officer from the College will discuss any requirements for additional assistance as required.

x. Guideline development group develops recommendations
(see also 3.10, 3.11)
This key stage will require a meeting of the guideline development group to discuss the appraisal outcomes and develop the recommendations. A research and development officer from the College will also attend this meeting.

xi. Complete draft guideline document agreed (see also 3.12)
Agreement of the content of a first complete draft should be reached by members of the guideline development group prior to consultation. The writing of the draft will be coordinated by the Editorial Lead to ensure consistency in writing style and to ensure it meets the College's appraisal and approval requirements.

If third party material is being used as a source of information, it must be fully referenced within the document. Use or copying of large amounts of material, including text and images, without the permission of the writer/publisher, is in breach of copyright law (please see Appendix 13 for further information on clearing permissions).

xii. Peer review (see also 3.13)

Following agreement of the complete draft, a minimum of two external peer reviewers will be requested to review the guideline. The request will be coordinated by the Project Lead and feedback shared with the Editorial Lead and the core guideline development group. A month should be allowed for feedback.

xiii. Consultation (see also 3.3, 3.4)

A copy of the complete agreed draft should also be distributed for consultation with key individuals or organisations, as outlined in the project plan for service user and stakeholder involvement. The distribution will be coordinated by the Project Lead and feedback shared with the Editorial Lead and the core guideline development group.

xiv. Revisions to complete draft

Feedback received from peer review and consultation should be reviewed by the group, responses agreed and documented, and the guideline amended accordingly.

At this stage the group should also apply for any external endorsements, approaches in relation to writing a foreword, permission to co-badge, etc.

DEVELOPMENT STAGE FLOWCHART

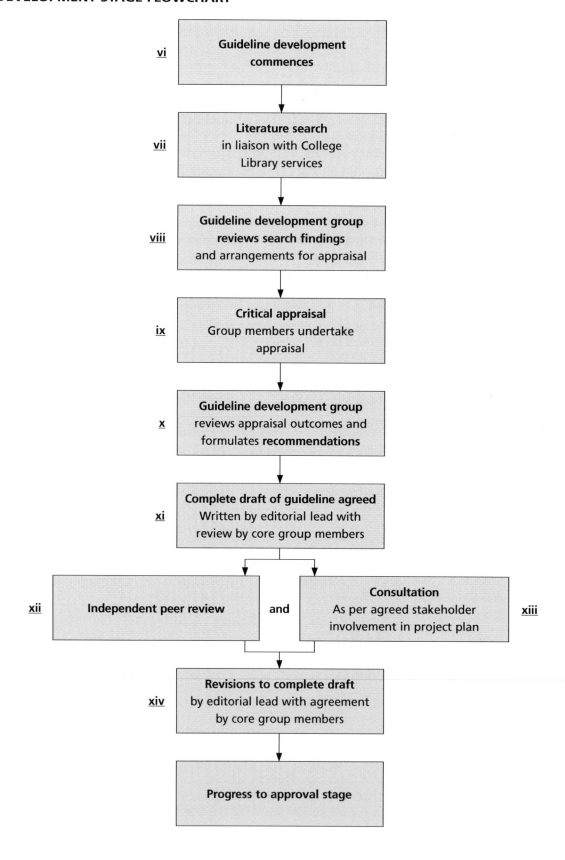

5.6 Approval and publication stage (3–4 months)

xv. Guideline draft submitted to the PPG

A revised complete draft of the guideline should be submitted to the PPG, together with stakeholder comments and the guideline development group's responses. The PPG will use the *AGREE II* tool (AGREE Next Steps Consortium 2013) as the assessment framework. The draft should be a comprehensive document, which is fully referenced (both within the text and within the reference list) and proofread. Incomplete text and missing references can significantly delay the publication process. If the document includes images or diagrams then these must be included, and evidence of any relevant permissions should also be submitted. Following evaluation of the guideline by the PPG, feedback will be sent to the Project Lead.

xvi. Editing of final agreed draft

Comments provided in response to the document submitted to the PPG should be used to guide the group in formulating a final agreed draft. This final draft will then be considered by the PPG and, if all criteria are met, will be approved. The group must ensure that all contributors are acknowledged and listed in this version. Once approved, and signed off by the College, the final draft will be handed over, via the College's Quality Programme Manager, to the College's Library for a full reference check.

xvii. Production

The College's Quality Programme Manager will liaise with the Publications Manager in order to manage the final stages through manuscript production to print. This will include copy-editing, typesetting, proofreading and front cover design. The College's Publications Manager will liaise with the Project and Editorial Leads, together with the Quality Programme Manager, to resolve any queries arising from the copy-edit and to finalise/check proofs.

During this stage the group must also finalise any necessary arrangements in relation to the storage of any data and documents (for example, search strategy and findings, conflicts of interest forms) that may have been generated as a result of developing the publication.

xviii. Promotional activities

On publication the guideline will be available for free download from the College website.

To ensure the guideline reaches all those for whom it is intended, the College will assist in the promotion and distribution of the guideline. This will be done in discussion with the Project Lead.

Occupational Therapy News (OTnews), the College website, flyers, email networks, social media and launches are just some of the ways to raise awareness of the guideline. It can also be beneficial to distribute a number of complimentary copies to relevant stakeholders and/or endorsing organisations.

All higher education institutions with occupational therapy programmes will be alerted to the publication, with a request that its availability is drawn to the attention of the students.

APPROVAL AND PUBLICATION STAGE FLOWCHART

xv

```
┌─────────────────────────────┐
│   Complete guideline draft  │◄──────────┐
│     submitted to the PPG    │           │
│  by editorial and project leads │       │
└─────────────────────────────┘           │
              │                    Further work
              ▼                    required
        ◇─────────────◇                │
       ╱  PPG approval?  ╲─────────────┘
        ◇─────────────◇        No
              │ Yes
              ▼
```

xvi

```
┌─────────────────────────────┐
│     Editing of final draft   │
│       and sign off by COT    │
└─────────────────────────────┘
              │
              ▼
```

xvii

```
┌─────────────────────────────┐
│          Production          │
└─────────────────────────────┘
              │
              ▼
```

xviii

```
┌─────────────────────────────┐
│     Promotional activities   │
└─────────────────────────────┘
```

5.7 Post-publication stage

The College recommends that practice guidelines should be updated within a maximum period of five years from publication or, if agreed, withdrawn. The scheduled review period may, however, need to be revisited if significant new evidence becomes available that could have an impact on the validity or appropriateness of the recommendations in a guideline.

xix. Evidence awareness

A 'handover brief' should be produced by the guideline development group at the end of a guideline project to facilitate the Specialist Section to monitor for pertinent new evidence within the guideline scope.

The National Executive Committee (NEC) of a Specialist Section, which has responsibility for a practice guideline published by the College of Occupational Therapists, should include an objective relating to that guideline(s) within their annual business plan.

The most appropriate member(s) of the National Executive Committee (e.g. Clinical Forum Lead, R&D Lead) is nominated to coordinate and record the 'evidence awareness' process.

A six-monthly alert system to identify publications using agreed search terms is coordinated by the College of Occupational Therapists Library and sent to the COT Research and Development Officer. References will be sent to the nominated Specialist Section NEC members for their review at least annually.

In cases where new evidence would potentially have an impact on the recommendation statements, a more formal review will need to be established.

xx. Guideline review group established

The scheduled review and updating process should commence prior to the identified review date (for example, up to two years before the five-year review date). This lead-in time is important to ensure adequate time for progressing a full review/development process where indicated.

The review group should consist, where possible, of one or more members of the original guideline development group. The Specialist Section, or group with responsibility for the guideline, should nominate/seek volunteers with the relevant skills and expertise to be members of the review group.

xxi. Identify new relevant evidence

The review group should use the results of an updated literature search to examine the relevant evidence published since the original guideline search date. Group representatives' knowledge of developments in the field should also be discussed.

Clinical trial databases may additionally be scanned to provide an indication of relevant research that may be published in the future, and which may influence the guideline scope.

xxii. Assess need for an update

New evidence should be considered in the context of the existing guideline content.

Key questions that the review group must consider are:

• Is any new evidence relevant to the original guideline scope?

• What impact would the new evidence have on existing guideline recommendations?

• Would the new evidence indicate the need for additional recommendations?

• If no new evidence, does the existing guideline still provide best available evidence to inform practice?

• Can the existing guideline be confidently followed as safe practice?

The needs assessment should include evaluation of feedback from occupational therapists and others with respect to the demand for, and the application of, the guideline.

xxiii. Guideline does not require updating

Where an assessment indicates that the existing guideline remains valid (i.e. no new relevant evidence and guideline recommendations remain safe and effective practice), then the outcome will be that the guideline should be reprinted.

The reprint must include:

• A statement in the section on 'Updating the guideline':
The guideline was reviewed in 20XX in line with the *Practice guideline development manual* (20XX) requirements. No new relevant evidence was identified. The guideline development group has assessed that the guideline, and its recommendations, continue to define the best available evidence to support effective practice.

• Date of review (when review outcome ratified).

• Date of next review (maximum of five years).

Guidelines that have been reviewed as scheduled, but the content unchanged, may be included on the website for up to a period of 10 years from the original date of publication.

All guidelines will be automatically withdrawn 10 years after the original publication date.

xxiv. Guideline requires updating

The updating process will reflect the main guideline development process.

All updating projects should include:

• Literature search (which, subject to any refinement, should replicate the original guideline search strategy and start from the date of the previous search).

• Appraisal of new evidence.

• Consideration of any original material that is no longer appropriate and how this might need to be superseded or withdrawn.

• Consideration of new evidence that reinforces existing recommendations.

• Consideration of any relevant feedback and comments received since the publication of the guideline.

• Development of recommendations where indicated by new evidence or knowledge.

The nature, strengths and weaknesses of new evidence identified will influence the extent of the updating process. Where there are significant changes in recommendations anticipated, then early engagement of stakeholders and service users will be indicated.

The updated guideline document should include:

• Details of the review/updating process followed, with relevant sections of the document updated as indicated.

• Clear annotation to identify where new recommendations have been included or existing recommendations have been revised/withdrawn.

• Date of review (when review outcome ratified).

• Date of next review (maximum of five years).

xxv. External review

If there are any new or amended recommendations indicated as a result of a review, consultation with stakeholders, service users and end users should be undertaken, together with external peer review.

xxvi. PPG ratification

The outcome of the review of any guideline (either remaining valid or subject to the updating process) must be submitted to the College of Occupational Therapists' Practice Publications Group for ratification.

xxvii. Publication

Updated or reprinted guidelines will be processed by the College's Publications Manager.

POST-PUBLICATION STAGE FLOWCHART

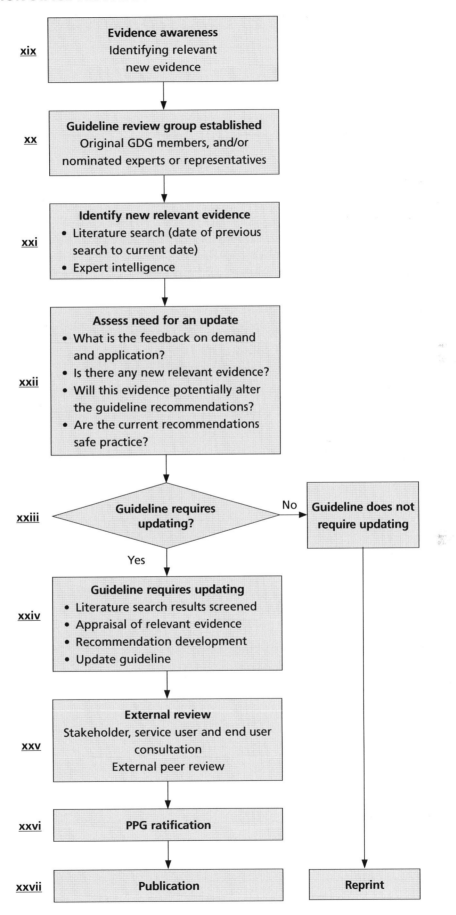

Appendix 1 Proposal form for the PPG

Practice Publications Group:
Proposal form

This form should be completed by any group that wishes to develop occupational therapy practice guidelines in partnership with the College of Occupational Therapists. You are advised to complete the form only after your advisory meeting with the College's Quality Programme and Research and Development Managers.

Points to consider before completing this form:

• Please ensure you have read the College's *Practice guideline development manual* (2017) prior to completing and submitting this form. In particular, you will be expected to have addressed all the points raised in section 3.1.

• In order for the College to make a decision about supporting and publishing your work, please provide as much detail as possible, as a lack of information could cause delays or result in the refusal of the request.

• Written approval for the guideline development project and confirmation of a funding amount from the Specialist Section Chair(s), or alternative source(s) as appropriate, must be submitted with this form.

• This proposal will be considered by the Practice Publications Group (PPG). This group meets three times a year (please refer to the College's website for the meeting dates) but proposals may be considered between meetings. Documents for approval by the PPG should be submitted to the College's Quality Programme Manager.

Organisation/Group name	
Contact name	
Contact address	
Postcode	
Telephone number	
Email address	
Signature and date	

1. OVERVIEW

1.1 Provisional guideline title

1.2 Please outline the practice guideline topic and its proposed overall objective

1.3 Outline how the topic will support an occupation-centred focus to practice

2. RATIONALE

Please refer to the College's Practice guideline development manual *section 3.1*

2.1 What need would this publication address?
Please include statistical information to support development, e.g. the prevalence of the condition, the population in question, etc.

2.2
(a) Who would this publication be relevant to? Who is/are your intended audience(s)?

(b) Who else might be interested in this document?

2.3
(a) How has it been established that there is a demand for occupational therapy practice guidelines in this particular area (what are the likely practice questions) at this particular time?

(b) How can you evidence this?

2.4 What national documents/strategies/policy drivers or care pathways does the proposed guideline link to?

2.5 Will the document be relevant UK-wide?
If not, please give reasons and indicate which countries it will cover, i.e. England, Northern Ireland, Scotland, Wales.

2.6 Following your initial literature searching and appraisal, please provide an outline of key evidence that exists to support practice guideline development in this area.

3. GUIDELINE DEVELOPMENT GROUP – SKILL MIX

Please refer to the College's Practice guideline development manual *sections 3.2, 3.3, 3.4 and 3.16*

3.1 Please provide the names of the core guideline development group members against the following individual backgrounds/skills:

- Expert practitioner
- Experience in developing professional documentation or writing skills *(this role can be fulfilled by a College Research and Development Officer)*
- Research experience (including critical appraisal)
- Project management experience
- Lay representatives
- Other stakeholder(s) (please state)

Please provide the names of those responsible for the following roles:

- Project lead
- Deputy Project Lead/Vice-Chair
- Editorial lead

3.2

(a) What other professional bodies or organisations have you approached to establish if they are engaged in similar work?

(b) If there is similar work being carried out, how would your document link with/complement it?

3.3 Please provide a list of stakeholders (e.g. professional bodies, charities, COT Specialist Sections) and lay representative organisations that have been contacted, and detail the expressions of interest received with regard to involvement in the guideline development project (this information can be provided as a separate table/attachment).

3.4 All guideline development group members must complete a declaration of conflicts of interest form before the project commences. Please state any declarations of conflicts of interest that have been identified at this stage that may impact on the development of this guideline topic.

4. MARKET CONTEXT

4.1

(a) Is this publication intended to replace an existing College document?

(b) If yes, give full details:

4.2

(a) What other published documents are there in the UK or abroad that are concerned with the same topic?

(b) If there are other documents (published or in development), what would the added value/impact of your proposed document be?

5. SUPPORT and FUNDING

Please attach details of secured funding.

5.1 Have ring-fenced funds been made available from the Specialist Section, or other sources, to support development, e.g. to buy in training/skills for the guideline development group, if necessary?   *Please state how much funding has been secured and submit written evidence with this form.*
5.2 Is funding available from potential collaborators?   *Please state how much funding has been secured and submit written evidence with this form.*   **Please note that all funding sources must be acknowledged and declared in the final document to ensure transparency.**

Please ensure you attach the required supporting paperwork (Q: 5) with your completed form and send to: Quality Programme Manager   Practice Publications Group   College of Occupational Therapists   106–114 Borough High Street   London SE1 1LB

For College use only:

Date

a) Proposal approved by PPG	Yes/No	
b) Decision deferred by PPG – request for further information	Yes/No	
c) Request approved by the College	Yes/No	

Publication request approved by Practice Publications Group (PPG)

Signature .... Date ....
Chair PPG

Publication request approved by College of Occupational Therapists

Signature .... Date ....
COT Assistant Director Professional Practice

Appendix 2 Scope form for the PPG

<table>
<tr><td colspan="2">

Practice Publications Group:

Scope form
</td></tr>
</table>

This form should be completed by any group that has received approval for their proposal to develop occupational therapy practice guidelines in partnership with the College of Occupational Therapists.

Please read and action as applicable the following before submitting this form:

• You must have submitted a publication proposal form to the Practice Publications Group (PPG) as part of the initial proposal stage and subsequently received approval to proceed to this stage.

• Please ensure you have read the College's *Practice guideline development manual* (2017) prior to completing and submitting this template.

• In order for the College to consider supporting and publishing your work, please provide as much detail as possible, as a lack of information could cause delays or result in the refusal of the request.

• Attach the **Stakeholder Information Document** [see Appendix 3] and additional material on further sheets if necessary, showing clearly the name of your organisation, guideline title and the number of the question in this template that the material relates to.

• At this stage, the PPG will be looking for evidence that the document will have an **occupation-centred focus**, be specific, unambiguous, unbiased, and that any health and wellbeing benefits will be balanced against possible risks and side effects.

• Note that approval at this stage means that the College is committed to supporting the development of this document. Publication of the final document will be subject to the manuscript meeting the College's quality standards. Support may be withdrawn at the College's discretion if the quality or progress of the document is deemed to be insufficient.

• **Please remember to attach a project plan/chart with detailed project milestones, timescales and envisaged costs.**

Organisation/Group name	
Contact name/telephone number	
Publication title	
Target audience	
Date	

> **Stakeholders are defined as follows:**
>
> • **Professional organisations and bodies:** e.g. other AHPs, RCN, social workers, charitable or third sector organisations, commissioners.
>
> • **Lay people:** i.e. individuals or organisations representing and/or supporting service users or carers.
>
> • **Service users and carers:** i.e. people who use or have used occupational therapy services.
>
> • **End users:** i.e. occupational therapists who will use the guideline.

1. SCOPE STAKEHOLDER INFORMATION DOCUMENT

The stakeholder information document includes sections on the overall objective of the guideline; the background; population and setting; and the practice question.

> **1.1 Please provide an outline of the stakeholder activities you have undertaken in the development of the scope, including details of the organisations, lay people, service users/carers and end users who participated (this information can be provided as a separate table/attachment).**
>
> *Ensure that you submit a Scope Stakeholder Information Document which should reflect the outcome of all scope development activity and consultation.*

2. EVIDENCE BASE

Please refer to the College's Practice guideline development manual *sections 3.7 and 3.8*

> **2.1**
> **(a) We appreciate that you will not yet have had access to a thorough literature search via the College Library, but please detail your knowledge of the evidence base to support the proposed publication.**
>
> **(b) What are the likely strengths and limitations of the evidence base, e.g. types of study and levels of evidence?**

> **2.2**
> **(a) Please list who will be leading on the critical appraisal of identified evidence, and the group members/co-opted others who will undertake appraisals.**
>
> **(b) Please confirm the critical appraisal framework you intend to use (either CASP or McMaster).**

2.3 Please describe your literature search strategy in terms of:

(a) Keywords for searching (list as many as possible for each aspect of your topic, giving synonyms, alternative English or American spellings or terminology, single and plural word forms, etc.). All searches will include terms to identify evidence on cost effectiveness and economic evaluation.

(b) The following databases will be routinely searched: AMED, CINAHL, HMIC, PsycINFO, OTSearch, OTDBASE, OTSeeker, the Cochrane Library, MEDLINE, Social Policy and Practice, and the COT Library Catalogue. If you are aware of any other specialist databases/resources, please give details below.

(c) Please specify the time period the search will cover (e.g. 10 years).

(d) Please provide any additional information which would help inform the literature search.

NB: Any handsearching of journals required will be the responsibility of the guideline development group.

3. GUIDELINE DEVELOPMENT GROUP

Please refer to the College's Practice guideline development manual *sections 3.2, 3.3, 3.4 and 3.12*

3.1 Confirm the membership of the core guideline development group (give names and affiliations).

3.2 Provide details of the stakeholders who will be involved in the guideline development during the course of the project, including at what stage, their role and contributions, etc. – this can be provided as a separate spreadsheet or table.

- Professional organisations/bodies:

- Lay people:

- Service users and carers:

- End users:

4. IMPLEMENTATION

Please refer to the College's Practice guideline development manual *section 4*

4.1 Detail any ideas that have been considered at this stage with respect to the possible range of tools to support implementation (other than the standard Quick Reference Guide, Audit Tool and Professional Development Resource).
4.2 Detail any additional/supporting information that you wish to submit.

Please ensure that you attach the required supporting paperwork (e.g. scope stakeholder information, project plan/chart) to your completed template and send to:

Quality Programme Manager
Practice Publications Group
College of Occupational Therapists
106–114 Borough High Street
London SE1 1LB

For College use only:

Date

a) Scope approved by PPG	Yes/No	
b) Decision deferred by PPG – request for further information	Yes/No	
c) Request approved by the College	Yes/No	

Publication request approved by Practice Publications Group (PPG)

Signature .... Date ....
Chair PPG

Publication request approved by College of Occupational Therapists

Signature .... Date ....
COT Assistant Director of Professional Practice

Appendix 3 Scope stakeholder information

Practice guideline scope stakeholder information

This document will provide the outline (scope) for the production of a practice guideline for occupational therapists working with [xxxx]. The guideline development work is being led by the College of Occupational Therapists Specialist Section – [xxxxx].

The guideline development group is aware that some stakeholders may be less familiar with the role occupational therapists have in relation to [xxxxx]; however, all contributions to the development of the final scope will be welcome and appreciated.

What is occupational therapy?

Occupational therapy enables people to achieve health, wellbeing and life satisfaction through participation in occupation (WFOT 2013, p48). 'Occupation' refers to practical and purposeful activities that allow people to live independently and have a sense of identity. This could be essential day-to-day tasks such as self-care, work or leisure (COT 2016).

Provisional guideline title

Practice need for the guideline

Background to the clinical condition/situation and associated national statistics

The occupational therapy role in this area of practice

Objective of the practice guideline

Practice question(s) to be addressed by the guideline

Population to be covered by the guideline (e.g. age range, gender, ethnicity, culture, condition, etc.)

Population or any groups that will not be covered by the guideline (with rationale for exclusion)

Setting in which the guideline will be applicable (e.g. community, hospitals, schools, etc.)

Key occupational therapy intervention(s) that the guideline will cover

Key occupational therapy intervention(s) that the guideline will not cover (with rationale for exclusion)

Key outcomes anticipated for service users/carers as a result of the occupational therapy intervention(s)

Any comparisons between the intervention(s) and other therapies or care – as applicable

How the guideline will support an occupation-centred focus to practice

Potential health inequalities and social determinants that need to be considered within the guideline (for example, best start in life for children; fair employment and good work for all; healthy standard of living for all; maximising individual capability and control over life; creating and developing healthy and sustainable places and communities; and strengthening the role and impact of ill-health prevention)

Anticipated impact of an occupational therapy practice guideline on this topic

References

College of Occupational Therapists (2016) *What is occupational therapy?* London: COT. Available at: *https://www.cot.co.uk/ot-helps-you/what-occupational-therapy*

World Federation of Occupational Therapists (2013) *Definitions of occupational therapy from member organisations*. Forrestfield, AU: WFOT. (This document can be accessed from the Resource Centre: filter resources by category 'General'). Available at: *http://www.wfot.org/resourcecentre.aspx*

[Insert references as applicable]

Thank you for considering this scope document.

A Scope Stakeholder Feedback Form is provided to record your comments and any conflicts of interest.

All comments need to be received by: XXXXXX

The feedback form and any questions about the project should be sent to the guideline Project Lead:

[Insert Project Lead details]

Email: XXXXX

Appendix 4 Appraisal tools

Different types of appraisal tool are generally tailored for different study types, but all facilitate the reviewer to appraise the evidence against areas, which typically include (depending on study type) the following: study purpose; literature review; design and its appropriateness; biases; sample/recruitment; intervention; data collection; data analysis; results/outcomes; ethical considerations; overall rigour; drop-outs; conclusions and clinical implications.

McMaster University evidence appraisal framework

The McMaster University framework has a specific occupational therapy focus and two tools with comprehensive guidance notes for:

• Quantitative review (Law et al 1998).

• Qualitative review (Letts et al 2007).

Critical Appraisal Skills Programme (CASP)

CASP has critical appraisal tools available for:

• Systematic reviews.

• Randomised controlled trials.

• Qualitative research.

• Economic evaluation studies.

• Cohort studies.

• Case control studies.

• Diagnostic test studies.

(These tools are copyright to CASP UK.)

The tools can be accessed, subject to copyright requirements, via the McMaster University or Solutions for Public Health websites respectively. Details of the tool(s) used and the relevant acknowledgement must be recorded in the guideline document.

Further details can be found at:

http://srs-mcmaster.ca/research/evidence-based-practice-research-group/

http://www.casp-uk.net/

Grey literature

Grey literature includes conference papers, theses/dissertations, conference papers and other reports. Grey literature can be evaluated/appraised using the AACODS checklist (Tyndall, J. (2010) *AACODS checklist.* Adelaide [Flinders University]. Available at: *http:// dspace.flinders.edu.au/jspui/bitstream/2328/3326/4/AACODS_Checklist.pdf)*

Appendix 5 Evidence tables template

Source	Design and participants	Intervention	Outcomes	Results	Quality and comment

Source	Design and participants	Intervention	Outcomes	Results	Quality and comment

Appendix 6 Recommendation decision table template

Key question/outcome	
Recommendation statement Detail the recommendation that the guideline development group makes from the evidence. Define strength of recommendation (1 = strong – 'It is recommended . . .' or 2 = conditional – 'It is suggested . . .')	**Strength of recommendation (1 or 2)**
Quality of evidence statement Summary of the synthesis of the evidence relating to the key question and overall evidence level (A = High, B = Moderate, C = Low, D = Very low)	**Overall quality of evidence level**
Evidence table references	
Quality and volume of evidence Are there any issues concerning the quantity of evidence available on this topic, its methodological quality and consistency?	
Generalisability How reasonable is it to generalise from the results of the studies used as evidence to the target population for this guideline?	
Applicability To what extent is the evidence directly applicable to occupational therapy in the UK?	
Clinical impact Due consideration should be given to the following: significance of the outcome, benefits and risks, financial barriers, organisational barriers, and any issues related to health inequalities or social determinants of health.	
Other factors considered by the guideline development group and any variance of opinion.	

Adapted from the 'Considered judgement form' (SIGN 2008) with permission from the Scottish Intercollegiate Guidelines Network.

Appendix 7 Guideline document template

A published guideline should normally include the following components, although the order in which the content appears may vary.

Contents

Foreword

Key recommendations for implementation

• This provides a summary of the guideline recommendations and their grading of quality and strength.

Introduction

• Practice requirement for the guideline.

• Topic identification process.

• Reference to national context and any other relevant publications.

• Context of service delivery/background to clinical conditions.

Occupational therapy role

Objective of the guideline

• Overall objective of the guideline.

Guideline scope

• Clinical, healthcare or social questions covered by the guideline.

• Population and target audience to whom the guideline applies.

Guideline recommendations and supporting evidence

• This contains the evidence information and consists of an introduction, details of evidence identified, quality of evidence, any discussion and interpretation and subsequent recommendation. This may be in sections related to the topic: for example, care pathway, themes, occupational domains, etc.

• Includes presentation of different options for management or intervention as appropriate.

• Reference is made to specific clinical, healthcare or social circumstances in which the guideline applies.

• Recommendations must consider/discuss the health benefits, side effects and any risk issues associated, and potential impact.

Service user/carer perspectives

Implementation of the guideline

• Includes details of any support tools, audit and review criteria.

• Discusses the potential organisational and financial barriers for the application of the recommendations.

Recommendations for future research

• Identifies the gaps in the evidence base and potential research priorities.

Guideline development process

• Guideline development group (how established, membership, end users).

• Stakeholder involvement.

• Service user involvement (how involved and in what aspects).

• External peer review and consultation (details of how this has taken place).

• Conflicts of interest.

• Declaration of funding for the guideline development.

• College appraisal and ratification process.

Guideline methodology

• Guideline question(s).

• Literature search strategy and outcomes (includes date of search).

• Criteria for inclusion and exclusion of evidence.

• Strengths and limitations of body of evidence and any uncertainty.

• Describes method used to arrive at recommendation (including any consensus activity).

• Identifies any limitations of the guideline and any potential bias in the conclusions or recommendations.

Updating the guideline

• Details when and how the guideline will be updated, with proposed date of review stated.

Appendices

Guideline development group

• Provides name, job title and name of institution or practice organisation.

Acknowledgements

• Details any other relevant contributors, stakeholders, service users, carers, peer reviewers, etc.

Conflicts of interest declarations (states any conflict of interest declared by guideline development group members, reviewers or stakeholders).

Literature search strategy

Evidence tables

Glossary and abbreviations

References

Appendix 8 Peer review proforma

Draft practice guideline – peer review proforma

Guideline title:	
Date for receipt of comments:	

Thank you for agreeing to be a peer reviewer for the above practice guideline.

Please critically appraise both the content and presentation of the guideline, taking into account the following areas and any others that you feel are pertinent, commenting as appropriate:

- Are the purpose and use of the guideline document adequately explained?

- Is the language used accessible and user-friendly?

- Is the text/terminology sensitive in terms of gender, race, culture, etc.?

- Are there any sections that are poorly structured, unclear or difficult to understand?

- Is the process of development of the guideline reported robust, explicit, transparent and unbiased?

- Is it explicit how the recommendations have been developed from the evidence?

- Are the recommendations and supporting evidence presented clearly?

- Is the text inclusive of all people who may use it, e.g. students, practitioners, educators, researchers?

- What is your overall view of the guideline document?

Detailed copy-editing comments are not expected, as the draft document will be edited before publication.

We require you to disclose any conflicts of interest (*identified as either a personal interest (of you, your partner or close relatives) or non-personal interest (of your department/employer/business), which could have the potential to influence or affect your contribution to the development or content of occupational therapy guidelines*), but if you have any concerns about whether a conflict of interest would preclude you from reviewing the document, please contact the Project Lead.

Your comments will be sent to the developers to inform the final draft, and acknowledgement of your contribution as a peer reviewer will be included in the published document.

Details of the College of Occupational Therapists' guideline development process, which is NICE Accredited, can be found in the College of Occupational Therapists' Practice guideline development manual (2017) *available at: http://www.cot.co.uk.*

We would be grateful if you could ensure that your comments are received by: ....

If you have any difficulty with this timescale, or have any questions, please contact:

[Name], Project Lead at: [email address]

On behalf of: [Name of College Specialist Section/regional/other group]

Draft practice guideline – peer review proforma

Guideline title:	
Date for receipt of comments:	

Please give your preferred details for acknowledgement in the published guideline:

Name	
Role	
Organisation	

Section of document	**Comment**

Please submit your comments electronically, together with a completed declaration of conflicts of interest form (located on the following page) to: ....

Appendix 9 Conflicts of interest declaration form

Practice guideline development conflicts of interest declaration
Guideline title:

The College of Occupational Therapists (COT) values your involvement in the development of practice guidelines for occupational therapists. To ensure that the guideline developed cannot be found to be biased, you must consider whether you may have any interests that may potentially conflict with the role you will be taking in the guideline development.

A conflict of interest is identified as either a personal (of the person, their partner or close relatives) or non-personal (of their department/employer/business) interest which could have the potential to influence or affect an individual's ability to act in the best interests of COT. Interests can be considered as either 'specific' or 'non-specific' in relation to the matter under discussion.

Type of interest	Description of interest (if you have no interests in a category, state 'none')
Involvement in research and published evidence in relation to the guideline topic.	*Nature of involvement and associated dates*
Involvement in the development of guidelines within this topic area for another organisation.	*Name of organisation, nature of involvement and associated dates*
Ordinary membership of professional bodies, Specialist Sections, committees, charities, voluntary bodies, etc.	*Name of body*
Office held in professional bodies, Specialist Sections, committees, charities, voluntary bodies, etc.	*Name of body and nature of office held*
Consultancies, research or other positions with any commercial companies with interests in the guideline topic area or which might potentially benefit from the guideline recommendations.	*Name of companies and position(s) and associated dates*
Other relevant interests that could lead to a perception of bias when giving opinions at any stage during the guideline development process.	

I hereby declare the above is an accurate declaration of my interests in relation to my current and anticipated involvement in the development of the above guideline:

Signature: ....

Name (*please print*): .... Date: ....

Job title: .... Employer: ....

A copy of the College's Conflicts of Interest Policy can be accessed on the website at: *http://www.cot.co.uk/policies*. Details specific to guideline development are included in the *Practice guideline development manual* available at: *https://www.cot.co.uk/practice-guidelines/practice-guidelines-development-process*.

Appendix 10 Management of conflicts of interest

Occupational therapists invited or volunteering to join a guideline development group are likely to be members of a College of Occupational Therapists' Specialist Section. Group members will, therefore, inevitably have some potential 'non-specific' conflict of interest by virtue of their professional interests (e.g. membership of clinical forums or specialist professional organisations) and expertise (e.g. practice specialists, researchers). Some individuals, by virtue of the relatively small pool of experts, may have more 'specific' conflicts (e.g. author of evidence, member of the Specialist Section National Executive Committee). Establishing whether individuals have any conflict of interest currently, or anticipated over the project timeline, enables the appropriate management of any interests during the guideline development activities and meetings.

All completed conflicts of interest forms should be kept by the Project Lead for the duration of the project, with copies sent to the College of Occupational Therapists' Quality Programme Manager.

Management of conflicts of interest: checklist

1 A conflicts of interest form must be completed by the proposed Project Lead and submitted to the College of Occupational Therapists' Quality Programme Manager for review. This is to ensure that there are no specific interests that may preclude the individual leading the project.

2 A conflicts of interest form must be completed by all invited or volunteering core guideline group members prior to commencement of, or involvement in, the guideline activity. Forms should be reviewed by the identified Project Lead with advice sought as required from the College of Occupational Therapists' Quality Programme Manager. This is to confirm that there is no specific conflict of interest which would preclude membership.

3 The guideline proposal form (Appendix 1) must include details of any potential conflicts of interest identified with regard to the group's members. This will be reviewed as part of the submission to the College of Occupational Therapists' Practice Publications Group. Where any concern is raised, clarification will be sought from the Project Lead.

4 A member of the group should be nominated to the role of Deputy/Vice-Chair.

5 Declarations of interest must be included as a standard agenda item for every meeting of the guideline development group. Group members must declare any conflicts in relation to the specific matters under discussion on the agenda for that meeting, or any changes since last completing the declaration form.

6 Where an interest is declared at a meeting, then it should be clarified if it relates directly to the matter under discussion. Where the interest is specifically relevant, the Project Lead/Chair, with the consensus of the rest of the guideline development

---

group members, will determine the most appropriate action to manage that interest, i.e.:

- Group member remains in the meeting but does not participate in discussion or any decision-making OR

- Group member remains in the meeting, participates in the discussion but not in the decision-making OR

- Group member withdraws from the meeting during the item under discussion and whilst any decision is made (action normally appropriate for any personal financial interest).

If the interest is not specifically relevant then, following declaration, participation should be feasible unless specific circumstances indicate otherwise.

If the conflict is with the Project Lead/Chair, then the nominated Deputy/Vice-Chair will lead the meeting, or agenda item, in line with one of the three options above.

7   Declarations of interest and actions taken to manage any conflict must be recorded in the meeting minutes.

8   A new conflicts of interest form will be completed annually by core group members in line with the College of Occupational Therapists' Conflicts of Interest Policy.

9   All abstracts for screening must be checked prior to allocation to ensure authors do not screen their own work.

10 All evidence for critical appraisal must be checked prior to allocation to ensure no authors appraise their own publications.

11 The Project Lead/Chair should ensure that all members have the opportunity to contribute their point of view in discussions during guideline development group meetings.

12 All co-opted members and peer reviewers will be asked to complete a conflicts of interest form.

13 Individuals participating in any guideline consultation activity will be asked to declare any conflicts of interest in writing or, if participating in a face-to-face consultation group activity, verbal declarations will be recorded by the group facilitator.

14 A clear statement outlining conflicts of interest, and declarations made, must be included within all published guidelines.

Appendix 11 The College's Practice Publications Group terms of reference

<u>Responsible to:</u> **COT Council** (via the Professional Practice Business Report)

1. ROLES

1.1 **Strategic:** To provide a quality assurance role in reviewing proposals and drafts produced by the College of Occupational Therapists' Specialist Sections, regional and other groups who wish to publish practice documents in collaboration with the College.

1.2 **Governance:** To ensure that all practice publications maintain a style and quality that supports the professional and public standing of the College of Occupational Therapists.

2. RESPONSIBILITIES

2.1 To review practice publication proposals, incorporating planned new work by COT Specialist Sections, new work in response to professional or national developments, and the review of published documents.

2.2 To support the development of agreed new work, through the provision of information, advice, templates and critical appraisal.

2.3 To ensure that proposals and draft manuscripts are assessed against the College's agreed evaluation criteria and, where applicable, NICE Accreditation criteria (NICE 2014).

2.4 To ensure that all publications are appropriate to the readership, whether UK-wide or country specific.

2.5 To support a consistent, reliable and timely publication process within the College.

2.6 To encourage and support collaborative multiprofessional development of publications that are relevant to allied health professions.

2.7 To ensure that information about the group and meeting dates are available on the College website, together with associated materials and briefings, to support members in the development of publications.

2.8 To involve and inform COT members, Council, boards and committees, and external interest groups, in the development of publications, as appropriate.

2.9 To report work progress and outcomes to the COT Council via the Professional Practice Business Report and the Quality Programme Manager.

2.10 The Chair and Quality Programme Manager will ensure that the UK COT Specialist Section Forum and relevant groups are informed of, and involved in, any publication issues of general interest and act as a communication link as required.

3. MEMBERSHIP

3.1 The membership will comprise:

3.1.1 **COT officers (3):**
Quality Programme Manager (Professional Practice)
Research and Development Manager (Education and Research)
Publications Manager (Communications and Marketing)

3.1.2 **Occupational therapy practitioners/managers (5):**
Five representatives from a range of health and social care backgrounds, with an interest in, and experience of, the production of professional documentation and evidence-based practice.

3.1.3 **Lay representatives (2):**
Two lay representatives with an interest in occupational therapy and improving health and social care, with a specific role of reviewing public-facing information.

3.1.4 **Co-opted members:**
One occupational therapist working in an educational/academic setting, with an interest and experience in the production of professional documentation and evidence-based practice.

3.1.5 **Experts** (usually one or two), with relevant knowledge and/or experience, may be co-opted to the group for the time taken to develop a particular publication.

4. RULES

4.1 A membership term will be three years. Vacancies will be advertised nationally.

4.2 The post of Chair will be held by a COT member, elected from the group. The Chair may delegate some tasks and authority to the appropriate College officers in order to progress the work of the group.

4.3 The Chair may be invited to attend COT board meetings when the agenda deems it necessary.

4.4 The Chair will be supported by a Vice-chair, also a COT member, elected from the group.

4.5 The posts of Chair and Vice-chair will not exceed their term of office. The out-going vice chair will normally become the subsequent chair.

4.6 A quorum shall be four members, one of whom must be the Chair or Vice-chair.

4.7 The group members who are occupational therapists must be members of COT.

4.8 Any member who fails to attend two consecutive meetings in any one year without providing a good reason, which is accepted by the group, may be deemed to have resigned. The Chair reserves the right to request further explanation or resignation where absence affects the business of the group.

4.9 When any member completes a term of office, one year should normally lapse before the member is eligible to apply and be considered for a further term of office.

5. MEETINGS

5.1 The PPG meets three times a year at the College of Occupational Therapists' headquarters in London.

5.2 The meetings are held in two sessions.

5.3 The first session looks at public-facing documents; the second session concentrates on membership materials. Group members will be required to undertake review of document submissions outside of the meetings.

6. ADMINISTRATION AND SUPPORT

6.1 The administration of the group will be carried out by a member of COT headquarters staff.

7. REVIEW DATE

7.1 Terms of reference to be reviewed three-yearly.

Conflicts of interest

Group members should declare any conflicts of interest at the beginning of a Practice Publications Group meeting or before the discussion of the item itself. These declarations and the actions that follow will be recorded in the minutes. Declaration forms should be completed and signed annually by all members of the group. The College's Conflicts of Interest Policy is available at: *www.cot.co.uk/policies*.

Appendix 12 College resources for guideline developers

Please note that the support and resources listed below are only available following approval of the guideline development project proposal by the PPG.

Resources, advice and support:

The College will provide:

• An initial advisory meeting with the College's Quality Programme Manager and College's Research and Development Manager.

• R&D Officer support at guideline development group meetings (see section 5 steps iv, vi, viii, x).

• Assistance with critical appraisal activities if required.

• Editorial Lead/co-lead role.

• Use of the College's meeting rooms free of charge (ensure booked as 'College guideline development project').

• Travel costs for group members (maximum of six) to attend up to four meetings per year over a two-year period.

• Travel/carer/childcare costs for lay representatives or service users (maximum of two) attending a guideline development meeting.

• Template forms (e.g. for stakeholder consultation of scope and draft guideline, and recording summary of stakeholder feedback).

• Advice and support during the development stage from the College's Quality Programme Manager.

• Advice and support during final manuscript to print stages from the Publications Manager.

• Front cover and document design.

• Safe and appropriate storage of any data and documentation.

College Library services:

For each guideline development project the College's Library will provide:

• Support from an information specialist to develop the subject search strategy and agree a set of terms for the literature search.

• One top-level evidence-based literature search (based on the agreed terms).

• Archiving of the search history to enable six-monthly evidence alerts following publication of the guideline.

• Free photocopying facilities for COT members undertaking work in collaboration with the College, i.e. group members may make single copies of publications held in the

Library for work relating to the development of guidelines. Photocopies are supplied in line with terms of the Copyright Licensing Agency (CLA) business licence. Group members may request copies of articles held in the Library for work relating to the development of guidelines, in line with the Library guidelines and terms. All reasonable photocopying requests will be met following discussion with the College Library and the Quality Programme Manager (NB the College Library can provide receipts for members to reclaim costs for photocopies and photocopy facilities). Copies of essential articles not held in the College can be ordered from the British Library in line with terms of the CLA business licence, i.e. group members may request copies of essential articles for work relating to the development of guidelines.

- Free personal use of the Library.

- Advice on referencing, including a copy of the College's referencing guidelines.

- One training session per publication on database searching for designated members of the group.

This service does not include the College Library borrowing materials from other libraries. Requests for such material will need to be made by group members to their host institutions.

Note that the CLA business licence allows members commissioned by the College to produce guidelines to make copies and request copies of articles for business purposes. However, every request to copy or order copies must made by an authorised member of the group. All requests for College Library services to support the production of guidelines should initially be made through the College's Quality Programme Manager. This is to ensure that a complete record of each guideline development project is kept on file and the Library can demonstrate that all copying has been undertaken in line with the terms of the CLA business licence.

The College Library offers one in-depth literature search per quarter to groups working on individual publications. Advance notice is required before the work can be undertaken and it needs to be scheduled in by the librarian. The Library will require a copy of the guideline development scope and prior detailed discussion with the Project Lead/subject expert to identify the search questions and specialist terminology.

Publishing services:

The College's communication and marketing team will provide:

- Production and printing services, covering all costs involved in producing hard copy documents when appropriate.

- An agreed number of complimentary hard copies for the development group/ contributors/Specialist Section forum (if applicable) to receive one copy each, plus copies for relevant outside agencies.

- Promotion of the published document in line with the College's publications marketing strategy.

- Reference copies of the final document for the College Library, higher education institutions (offering occupational therapy programmes), and legal deposit libraries.

- Notification to Nielsen to feed into online booksellers, and the British Library's Cataloguing in Publication (CIP) programme (an alerting service for libraries).

Appendix 13 Guideline development group responsibilities

Preparation

Members of the guideline development group should:

- Be aware of the requirements within the *Practice guideline development manual* as this will be used to form the framework and shape the guideline development process.

- Communicate with relevant College Specialist Sections/regional groups and/or other professional bodies regarding stakeholder involvement/collaboration in the guideline development project.

- Carry out initial literature searches to ensure there is a sufficient evidence base on which to base practice guidelines.

Funding

As explained in Appendix 12, travel costs for the guideline development group to attend meetings will be met by the College. However, the guideline development group is responsible for:

- Securing ring-fenced funding from the Specialist Section committee, and/or alternative sources, to cover any further development costs or for additional group member travel or expenses.

- Providing the College with written evidence of ring-fenced funds. In the event of the guideline development group having to buy in training/skills at any stage of the guideline development, the ring-fenced funds should be used to meet these costs.

Guideline development group

The guideline development group should:

- Agree on the appropriate skill mix and each member's specific role and division of responsibility within the group.

- Consider the time commitment this work involves before agreeing to be a member of the group.

- Complete and update as necessary all conflicts of interest forms and adhere to the guidance on conflict management (Appendices 9 and 10)

- Ensure that an agenda and minutes, recording all decisions and actions, are produced for each guideline development group meeting.

- Follow the development process, as explained in this manual, so that this is evident in the final guideline.

- Arrange room bookings (College or other) for guideline development group meetings.

Time management

It is the responsibility of the guideline development group to:

- Provide the PPG with a detailed action plan, including key stages of development and associated deadlines.
- Return requested paperwork/forms and respond to all PPG communications within the designated timeframes.

Communication

The group should agree:

- A commitment by all project members to meet timescales.
- An identified key link with the College, usually the Project Lead, with others prepared to assume responsibility if necessary.
- A plan for providing quarterly updates to the College Quality Programme Manager to help keep momentum and maintain motivation.
- A mechanism for advising the College immediately of any risk to the scheduled handover of the final draft to the College in line with the action plan, e.g. change in membership of group, slippage to timescales, etc.
- A plan for arranging peer review of the draft guidelines.
- An action plan for engaging and consulting with stakeholders, and for approaching external organisation(s) regarding the provision of a foreword and/or endorsement of the final document.

Permissions and approvals

The guideline development group is responsible for:

- Seeking permission to use third party material and providing written evidence of clearance where necessary. Refer to the COT Briefing 101 on *Copyright* for further information (*www.cot.co.uk/research/briefing-101-copyright*) and see also Appendix 14.
- Adhering to any relevant research governance/project ethics requirements.
- Complying with the College's requirements in relation to any data and documentation storage (additional guidance available).

Implementation and evaluation

Developers share responsibility with the College for the promotion and implementation of the published guideline.

Developers should also undertake evaluation activities to determine the impact of the guideline and help inform future review.

Review

The guideline development group is responsible for the review of the practice guideline in line with the handover brief mentioned in section 5.7 of this manual.

Appendix 14 Copyright

The letter of agreement that the guideline development group will be asked to sign, if the publication request is approved, includes assignment of copyright to the College. This gives the College the right to publish the document and also enables the College to manage any permission and translation requests on the group's behalf (i.e. requests from others to use extracts from your work in their own publications or to distribute translated versions). It also allows the College to:

- Make editorial corrections to the submitted material (NB the guideline development group will have a chance to see and comment on first proofs).

- Publish the material in any form or medium (primarily hard copy and web download), including extracts, e.g. for marketing purposes.

- Allow third party publication of the material where appropriate (e.g. via the NICE Evidence database).

- Distribute and sell the publication worldwide.

- Translate the material or grant permission to translate (e.g. for Welsh speakers).

- Adapt and update the material if appropriate (NB where possible this will be via the original guideline development group or, where necessary, alternative members of the relevant Specialist Section).

- Take steps to deal with breaches of copyright (i.e. illegal use of the material by third parties).

Please note that the guideline development group will not be able to:

- Publish the material itself or via another third party (including online or in hard copy) without agreement from the College.

- Publish or distribute extracts of the material*, distribute translations or give permission to others to do so (all requests should come via the College).

- Produce material itself or via another publisher on the same or similar topic as the agreed publication (which could adversely affect sales/downloads of the publication).

- Adapt/update the work or produce a new edition without the permission of the College (although note that agreement to publish this edition does not imply automatic agreement to produce all future editions).

* This applies to material over and above the amount permitted by copyright law. The College does allow use of the material in educational presentations. Whilst permission to use extracts of the material in other publications that the guideline development group may produce is unlikely to be refused, the College does ask that it is approached first as permission is granted on a case-by-case basis and the College also likes to keep track of all uses of published material.

Appendix 15 Summary chart of key stages of guideline development

(Full details of each stage are set out in Section 5.)

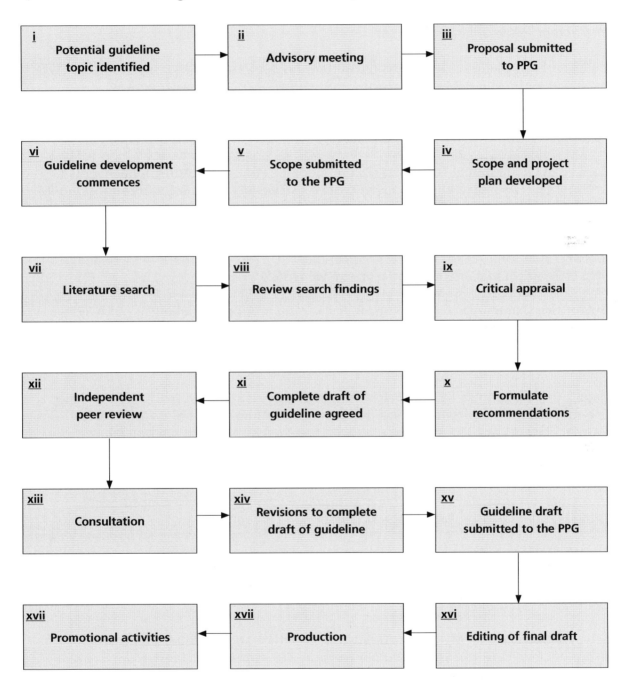

References

AGREE Next Steps Consortium (2013) *Appraisal of guidelines for research and evaluation II (AGREE II) instrument.* [s.l.]: The AGREE Research Trust. Available at: *http:// www.agreetrust.org/wp-content/uploads/2013/10/AGREE-II-Users-Manual-and-23-item-Instrument_2009_UPDATE_2013.pdf*

College of Occupational Therapists (2016) *What is occupational therapy?* London: COT. Available at: *https://www.cot.co.uk/ot-helps-you/what-occupational-therapy*

College of Occupational Therapists (2015a) Policy on conflicts of interests. London: COT. Available at: *https://www.cot.co.uk/policies*

College of Occupational Therapists (2015b) Code of ethics and professional conduct. London: COT. Available at: *https://www.cot.co.uk/sites/default/files/publications/public/ CODE-OF-ETHICS-2015.pdf*

GRADE Working Group (2004) Grading quality of evidence and strength of recommendations. [Online] *British Medical Journal, 328(7454),* 1490–1494. Available at: *http://www.ncbi.nlm.nih.gov/pmc/articles/PMC428525/*

Guyatt GH, Oxman AD, Vist GE, Kunz R, Falck-Ytter Y, Alonso-Coello P . . . GRADE Working Group (2008a) GRADE: an emerging consensus on rating quality of evidence and strength of recommendations. [Online] *British Medical Journal, 336(7650),* 924–926. Available at: *http://www.ncbi.nlm.nih.gov/pmc/articles/PMC2335261/*

Guyatt GH, Oxman AD, Kunz R, Falck-Ytter Y, Vist GE, Liberati A . . . GRADE Working Group (2008b) Going from evidence to recommendations. [Online] *British Medical Journal, 336(7652),* 1049–1051. Available at: *http://www.ncbi.nlm.nih.gov/pmc/articles/ PMC2376019/*

Health and Care Professions Council (2013) *Standards of proficiency: occupational therapists.* London: HCPC. Available at: *http://www.hpc-uk.org/assets/documents/ 10000512Standards_of_Proficiency_Occupational_Therapists.pdf*

Law M, Stewart D, Pollock N, Letts L, Bosch J, Westmorland M (1998) *Guidelines for critical review form: quantitative studies.* Ontario: McMaster University. Available at: *http://srs-mcmaster.ca/wp-content/uploads/2015/04/Guidelines-for-Critical-Review-Form-Quantiative-Studies-English.pdf*

Letts L, Wilkins S, Law M, Stewart D, Bosch J, Westmorland M (2007) *Guidelines for critical review form: qualitative studies (version 2.0).* Ontario: McMaster University. Available at: *http://srs-mcmaster.ca/wp-content/uploads/2015/05/Guidelines-for-Critical-Review-Form-Qualitative-Studies.pdf*

Marmot M (2010) *Fair society healthy lives: the Marmot review.* London: Marmot Review. Available at: *http://www.instituteofhealthequity.org/projects/fair-society-healthy-lives-the-marmot-review*

National Institute for Health and Care Excellence (2015) *Into practice guide.* (NICE Process PMG 30). London: NICE. Available at: *https://www.nice.org.uk/process/pmg30/ chapter/introduction-and-background#*

National Institute for Health and Care Excellence (2014) *Process manual for accrediting producers of guidance and recommendations for practice: a guide for producers and stakeholders.* London: NICE. Available at: *http://www.nice.org.uk/Media/Default/About/ accreditation/nice-accreditation-process-manual.pdf*

National Institute for Health and Clinical Excellence (2007) *How to change practice: understand, identify and overcome barriers to change.* London: NICE. Available at: *http://www.nice.org.uk/Media/Default/About/what-we-do/Into-practice/Support-for-service-improvement-and-audit/How-to-change-practice-barriers-to-change.pdf*

Pawson R, Boaz A, Grayson L, Long A, Barnes C (2003) *Types and quality of knowledge in social care.* (Knowledge Review 3). London: Social Care Institute for Excellence. Available at: *http://www.scie.org.uk/publications/knowledgereviews/kr03.pdf*

Richardson WS, Wilson MC, Nishikawa J, Hayward RS (1995) The well-built clinical question: a key to evidence-based decisions. *ACP Journal Club, 123(3),* A12.

Sackett DL, Straus SE, Richardson WS, Rosenberg W, Haynes RB (2000) *Evidence based medicine: how to practice and teach EBM.* 2nd ed. London: Churchill Livingstone.

Shekelle P, Woolf S, Grimshaw JM, Schünenmann HJ, Eccles MP (2012) Developing clinical practice guidelines: reviewing, reporting, and publishing guidelines; updating guidelines; and the emerging issues of enhancing guideline implementability and accounting for comorbid conditions in guideline development. [Online] *Implementation Science, 7:62.* Available at: *http://implementationscience.biomedcentral.com/ articles/10.1186/1748-5908-7-62*

Scottish Intercollegiate Guidelines Network (2008) *SIGN 50: a guideline developer's handbook.* Edinburgh: SIGN. Available at: *http://www.sign.ac.uk/pdf/sign50.pdf*

Tyndall, J. (2010) *AACODS checklist.* Adelaide [Flinders University]. Available at: *http:// dspace.flinders.edu.au/jspui/bitstream/2328/3326/4/AACODS_Checklist.pdf.*

Woolf S, Schünenmann HJ, Eccles MP, Grimshaw JM, Shekelle P (2012) Developing clinical practice guidelines: types of evidence and outcomes; values and economics, synthesis, grading, and presentation and deriving recommendations. [Online] *Implementation Science 7:61.* Available at: *http://implementationscience.biomedcentral. com/articles/10.1186/1748-5908-7-61*

World Federation of Occupational Therapists (2013) *Definitions of occupational therapy from member organisations.* Forrestfield, AU: WFOT. (This document can be accessed from the Resource Centre, filter resources by category: 'General'). Available at: *http:// www.wfot.org/resourcecentre.aspx.*

All websites in these references were accessed on 04.11.16.